MULTIHOSPITAL SYSTEMS

Multihospital Systems
The Process of Development

Diana Barrett

*Harvard School of
Public Health*

Oelgeschlager, Gunn & Hain, Publishers, Inc.

Cambridge, Massachusetts

International Standard Book Number: 0-89946-011-9

Library of Congress Catalog Card Number: 79-26111

Printed in the United States of America

Library of Congress Cataloging in Publication Data

Barrett, Diana.
    Multihospital systems.

    Bibliography: p. 171
    Includes index.
    1. Multihospital systems.   2. Multihospital systems
—United States.   I. Title.
RA971.B28   362.1'1   79-26111
ISBN 0-89946-011-9

Dedication

This book is dedicated to three groups of people, all of whom encouraged my interest in the development of multihospital systems: first of all, to the seven chief executive officers of the systems described herein; second, to the managers who have attended our program on multi-institutional collaboration at the Harvard School of Public Health; and finally, with great appreciation, to my family.

Contents

List of Figures and Tables

Figures

Tables

MULTIHOSPITAL SYSTEMS

Chapter 1

Evolution of the Research Topic

DEFINITION OF THE PROBLEM

The health system in the United States consumes growing proportions of our national resources, and it is not as consistent in quality or accessibility as one might wish. While economists, policymakers, and administrators are readily able to pinpoint the problems, they take issue with most proposed solutions, and cannot agree on what might be done to improve the health delivery system.

The multihospital system has emerged as a partial solution to some of these problems.[1] The term is commonly used to describe a formal or informal collaborative arrangement among two or more institutions. These systems can be local or regional. They can be horizontal—systems in which all the participating institutions provide similar care—or they can be vertically integrated—systems in which a variety of care is provided, including, for example, acute and long-term convalescent care. They can be profit-making or nonprofit systems. Forms of cooperation are varied and will be addressed in detail in Chapter 2, but it is important to define how the term "multihospital system" will be used in this book: it refers to a system in which a number of separate institutions are under a single corporate management that has overall authority for operating decisions and for policy formulation.

The development of multihospital systems is not a new phenomenon.[2] Indeed, this form of organization is but a more sophisticated evolution of the type of affiliation that has been in existence at least since World War II. As long ago as 1965, the Duke Forum, an annual conference held at Duke on various hospital related issues addressed the issue, and pressure certainly existed on hospitals for many years before that to combine their resources. Only recently, however, have pressures grown to the point that it is often imperative rather than optional to establish such systems.

There are approximately 350 systems in the United States and countless other arrangements in which hospitals work together on an ad hoc basis[3] (see Table 1.1).

In the exploratory research that led to this work, it became clear that while multihospital systems were emerging throughout the country, managers were taking all too little advantage of the data base formed by the experiences of the various systems. Few managers understood what was really similar or different among the different types, let alone what could be learned from the accumulated experience. While one system focused on financial problems, another allocated the major part of its management's time to civil rights issues. While one system seemed to have given considerable attention to the issue of membership, another appeared to be much concerned with improving the kind and the quality of care in a given geographical area.

Articles and research reports on the growth of multihospital systems seldom addressed the process of their development[4]—they seemed to assume that two or more institutions simply decided to "work together," and a system was thereby established. That is not to say that the research was vacuous; for example, the economic studies of system

Table 1.1. **A Summary of 1975 AHA Surveys of Multihospital Systems**

	1973	*1975*
Number of all hospitals in multihospital systems	845	1405
Number of proprietary hospitals in multihospital systems	193	309
Number of government hospitals in multihospital systems	101	309
Number of not-for-profit hospitals in multihospital systems	551	940
Multihospital system hospitals as percentage of all hospitals	15%	25%

Source: American Hospital Association, Chicago, Illinois, 1975.

effectiveness are certainly worthwhile—for it is clearly important to understand why some systems are more financially effective than others. But the research about the process leaves much unsaid—especially why and under what conditions systems develop, or falter, or fail. This research attempts to fill this gap.

The data base for the study consists of a sample of mature systems whose chief executive officer was interviewed. A preliminary model is developed that views the multihospital system as a product of its immediate environment and identifies aspects of the environment that are critical to the assurance of future growth.

ORGANIZATION OF THE BOOK

When I first considered multihospital systems (MHS) as a topic that I wished to pursue, an experienced hospital administrator expressed a view that no viable hospital would consider giving up its independence. I would argue that the concept of "viability" when it comes to hospitals is rapidly changing, and that the impact of the health system as a whole must be understood before the role of the MHS can be understood. For perspective, Chapter 2 places the MHS within the context of the system that provides health and illness care. The origin of the phenomenon is discussed by exploring the major problems within the health field that led to the development of the multihospital system.

The book is written from various perspectives and should be of interest to managers who are part of a system, to managers who are considering becoming part of a system, and also to researchers in the field of hospital administration. The early chapters, especially the second, should be of special value to the reader who is particularly interested in the changes in the health delivery system and in the environment in which it operates that have led to the formation of multihospital systems. The third and fourth chapters should be of special value to those readers who are interested in methodology and in the literature that pertains to hospital systems. The rest of the book is aimed at a broader audience—an audience of practical managers who want to learn from the history of other systems and from the experience of other managers. The later chapters consider those environmental factors that are particularly relevant to the development of an MHS, and in Chapter 7 the responses to external demands are presented. In Chapter 8 the role of the chief executive officer within an MHS is explored in order to better understand the importance of the linkages between the system itself and its environment. In Chapter 9, the conclusions are presented; in this chapter an exploratory model is developed which presents four hypotheses and proposes to link them in a way that can be used by both present and potential MHS administrators as well as by researchers. Chapter 10 addresses the implications of this research.

The reader will note that the case studies have been fictionalized because of the sensitivity of some situations and because the CEOs have a right to their privacy. Even though I obtained much of the material from public sources, the conclusions drawn are my own and hence subjective.

NOTES

1. The accepted name for this increasingly common organizational form is "multihospital system." Inasmuch as there are a variety of institutions represented in these systems besides hospitals, the term "multifacility system" would appear more appropriate. However, since the first term is accepted among administrators and researchers who have studied this phenomenon, I will refer to all sites as multihospital systems.
2. As of 1977, approximately 42 percent of hospital beds are part of a system.
3. Between 1973 and 1975, for example, the growth in the ratio of multihospital systems to all community short-term general hospitals reflects a two-thirds increase in just two years. The most significant growth occurred in the not-for-profit community hospitals, which have increased at over 35 percent per year, and all indications are that this rate of growth is continuing. (AMA survey of 1975)
4. See Chapter 4 for the review of relevant literature on Multihospital Systems.

Chapter 2

The Origin of the Phenomenon

INTRODUCTION

The U.S. health care industry has been described as the "fastest growing failing business in the world,"[1] a system that fails to meet the needs of many Americans.

The medical marketplace is today characterized by a number of conditions that cause it to deviate substantially from private industry. An understanding of the most important of these distinguishing characteristics is essential to an informed consideration of current problems in the health sector, as well as to an understanding of the role that the MHS can play in mitigating some of these problems. Following are the key distinguishing traits of the medical market that have direct impacts on the delivery of services:

Most consumers, represented by a third-party insurance provider—such as Medicare, Medicaid, Blue Cross–Blue Shield, or a commercial insurance carrier—are severed from the cost consequences of their consumption. The incentive to reduce costs does not come from the recipient of care.

There are substantial entry barriers in the health field, such as certificate of need, facility and personnel licensure, and heavy capital requirements. These barriers inhibit normal competitive pressures.

The complexity of modern medicine is such that consumers have relatively poor information about their needs and alternatives, and must rely heavily on providers of care to determine their demand for it. Again, this dampens the consumer's effectiveness in shaping the nature and cost of the product.

The delivery of some types of medical care, such as vaccinations, involves substantial externalities (e.g., benefits accrue not only to the people who receive medical attention, but also to those who come into contact with them). These externalities cause governmental subsidization, which again circumvents the working of the normal marketplace.

The predominance of cost-based reimbursement for hospital care removes the incentives for hospitals to reduce their costs.

Ninety percent of all hospital beds and most health care organizations are voluntary, nonprofit organizations. Consequently, the size of the institution, the range of services, teaching affiliation, and other noneconomic objectives have become increasingly important as indicators of performance.

Thus, the health care market is different from the normal for-profit market, and these differences have caused the problems that beset the health care system. The specific factors that have contributed to the development of multihospital systems are the following:

inflow of funds from third-party payers
excess hospital capacity
rising costs
changes in capital financing
changes in consumers' and physicians' expectations concerning the
   role of the hospital

These categories are not comprehensive, nor are they mutually exclusive; it is difficult to discuss changes in the capital structure without discussing changes in consumer expectations about the services that a hospital should make available. For purposes of simplicity, however, each factor and its impact on the development of multihospital systems will be addressed separately.

The second part of the chapter will summarize planning efforts that have represented a major attempt to rationalize the way in which health care is delivered. Finally, the multihospital system, a phenomenon that represents a major solution to the aforementioned problems, will be addressed.

FACTORS THAT HAVE LED
TO THE DEVELOPMENT OF
MULTIHOSPITAL SYSTEMS

Inflow of Funds from Third-party Payers

Approximately 60 percent of all hospital expenses are reimbursed through the cost-based formulas of Medicare, Medicaid, and Blue Cross. Although there are differences among these programs (particularly among the various Blue Cross plans), all are based on the principle of reimbursing "reasonable" and "allowable" costs incurred by hospitals. In practice, virtually all incurred hospital costs have been treated as allowable costs. Therefore, since reimbursement has been largely guaranteed, few hospitals have been motivated to make genuine efforts to contain costs. The preoccupation of American consumers and providers with curative, rather than preventive, medicine—and particularly with expensive new "miracle" procedures and technologies—has helped fuel the rise in hospital costs.

In Massachusetts, 35 to 40 percent of annual hospital revenues come from Medicare, 30 to 35 percent come from Blue Cross, 12 to 15 percent come from Medicaid, and the remaining 10 to 15 percent come from commercial carriers and out-of-pocket consumer payments. This significant inflow of funds from third-party payers reduced the percentage of health care costs paid directly to providers by patients from 80 percent in 1950 to 33 percent in 1976.[2] In the case of hospital care, the shift away from direct payment has progressed to the point that only about 9 percent of payments to hospitals in 1976 were made "out-of-pocket." This change in payment structure loosened what might otherwise have been a binding constraint on expenditure growth—the individual's ability to pay for the costs of increased technology, more qualified staff, and greater use of ancillary services. Consequently, the costs of hospital care continue to rise dramatically. Today, the perceived need for sophisticated services still exists, and even small community hospitals are attempting to provide a full range of services. Multihospital systems represent one way in which hospitals can provide these broad services to maintain their "attractiveness" to consumers and simultaneously reduce duplication, and therefore costs.

Excess Hospital Capacity

The economic and financial dynamics just discussed have had a number of impacts on the distribution, quality, and cost of health services. As costs have continued to climb, public comment has increasingly turned to specific problems in the delivery of acute inpatient services.

The phenomenon of the "excess" hospital bed has received much attention in recent years. Independent reports by Interstudy, the Institute of Medicine, the Public Citizen's Health Research Group, the Hill–Burton program, and a variety of regional and state planning bodies have concluded that we are oversupplied with hospital beds. The American Hospital Association has publicly recognized the need to trim the nation's bed complement.

Reducing Excess Hospital Capacity, a report issued by Interstudy in 1976, makes a useful distinction between "under-utilized hospital capacity" and "excessively-utilized hospital capacity."[3] Although the report includes ancillary services in the definitions of excess capacity, this discussion will focus on hospital beds. The report talks about underutilized capacity as capacity built, equipped, and staffed to provide a volume of services in excess of its actual utilization. Excessively utilized capacity is capacity used to provide inpatient services when alternative services of equal medical acceptability but lower intensity could have been supplied on an inpatient or ambulatory basis. Examination of each of these types of excess hospital capacity will help clarify the origins of bed oversupply estimates.

Researchers have based most of their conclusions regarding the existence of a hospital bed surplus on scrutiny of various utilization measures. These measures support the existence of both underutilized and excessively utilized capacity in the hospital sector.

As illustrated in Table 2.1, the number of community hospitals in the United States increased slightly, from 5,736 to 5,857, over the 1965–1976 period (see Table 2.1). During the same years, the number of beds in those hospitals increased sharply, from 741,000 to 956,000, or 29 percent, and the number of admissions exhibited a parallel growth, from 26,463,000 to 33,979,000, or 28.4 percent.

Table 2.1. Selected Measures in U.S. Community Hospitals, 1965–1976

Measure	1965	1976	Percent Change, 1965–1976
Hospitals	5,736	5,857	2.1
Beds	741,000	956,000	29.0
Admissions	26,463,000	33,979,000	28.4

Source: Hospital Statistics, copyright American Hospital Association, 1977.

These changes in the numbers of beds and admissions increase costs to the extent that the principal focus of public discussion of health care costs has been on the cost of hospital services.

There is little doubt that excess hospital capacity exists. However, it is often difficult to reduce this capacity because certain services are felt to be required by the community regardless of how often or seldom they are used. This is particularly true in geographically isolated areas where a consumer would indeed be inconvenienced by significant travel. The existence of a multihospital system allows cross-subsidization—a portion of the costs of these less profitable services to be absorbed by those that are more profitable, and by the effects of

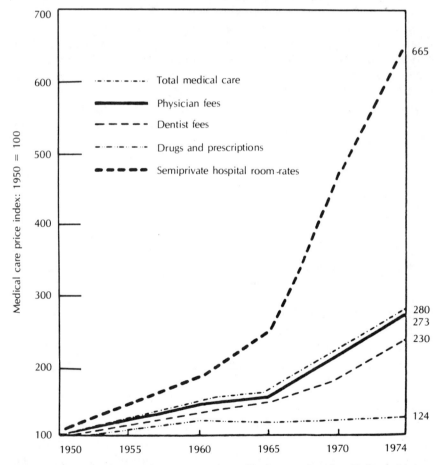

Figure 2.1. The increasing costs of medical care in the United States, 1950–1974.

operating a larger institution. While Certificate of Need and other measures meant to reduce and eliminate new building in order to reduce capacity have been proposed and enforced, the main problem with this approach is that such legislation affects new construction but does little to affect the ongoing operation. The MHS represents one way by which institutions can stabilize and strengthen ongoing operations rather than focus on the acquisition and building of new facilities.[4]

Rising Costs

There has been a significant shift since World War II in the demand for hospital services due to a growing population, progress in medical science, and rising social expectations. There were insufficient capital funds to meet this need; consequently, the government intervened by enacting the Hill–Burton Act to establish and expand hospitals in medically needy areas. The program provided up to two-thirds of the hospital's capital need; the matching restriction on these grants encouraged a greater flow of voluntary contributions and also precipitated the use of borrowing. Average daily charges began to increase rapidly during this period; inflation and the addition of education and community service programs contributed to increases in expenditures.[5]

One of the major issues is that incentives are created to increase rather than decrease costs and that, consequently, costs do rise. Consumers, for example, are in a very real sense isolated from the economic consequences of health care decisions since they pay little out-of-pocket for care and have little to say about what kind of care they should receive and what level of technical sophistication is necessary for a given diagnosis. Physicians, other than consumers, are the primary decisionmakers. They decide whether to hospitalize the patient, how long the patient will stay, which tests are to be ordered, and which procedures are to be followed. Traditionally, physicians have thought of care not in terms of costs but only in terms of quality, and quality has in turn been associated with larger and more "complete" facilities, which, of course, were more expensive. Thus, the physician and the patient act in a manner that is clearly in the physician's best interest and sometimes in the patient's best interest, but the cost of the care seldom affects their behavior.[6]

Costs have increased because it is more expensive to deliver care— particularly the kind of care that is considered acceptable today. Labor costs represent approximately 60 percent of a hospital's budget, and while hospital workers were once drastically underpaid, the 1960s witnessed an expansion of minimum wage requirements and unionization of hospital and health workers so that their salaries might "catch up" to those of workers in similar jobs in other industries. While the registered nurse earned $92.23 weekly in 1963, in 1969 the weekly wage had increased to $151.92.[7]

Hospital wages continue to rise more rapidly than any other wages in the economy. In the 1966–1975 period, hospital wages rose 8.7 percent each year while the earnings of all private nonagricultural workers increased 5.8 percent. There is no indication that the overall mix of hospital employers changed in the direction of higher skills and higher wages. If anything, the data imply that the number of employees with relatively low pay has grown faster than the number of more highly paid employees.[8]

Acceptable care usually means complex services using expensive new technology. Between 1965 and 1970, the percentage of hospitals with intensive care units increased almost 20 percent; those with physical therapy increased 10 percent. The most well-publicized example of this diffusion of extraordinarily expensive technology with little thought to utilization is the CAT scanner.[9] It is astounding, in fact, what the effect has been on hospital costs of increased salaries, technology, energy rates, and other factors. "Hospital prices—the prime propellant in health care inflation—are now nine times what they were in 1950; even after adjustment for general inflation, they are still nearly quadruple their 1950 level."[10] In fact, between 1965 and 1975, when the consumer price index rose 71 percent, the cost of the average hospital stay more than tripled, from $311 to $1,017, and during that period, the average length of stay actually decreased. During 1975 alone, the price of a semiprivate room rose 14.7 percent, and the average revenue per patient-day jumped 18.4 percent.[11] Hospital service charges continue to outpace increases in the Bureau of Labor Statistics Consumer Price Index listing for most other consumer goods and services. In February 1978, despite the voluntary effort of health care providers to slow the inflation rate, Labor Department figures showed a 1.3-percent increase for the "hospital and other medical services" index listing. This would come to about 14 percent on an annualized basis.[12]

This is not to say that the product that the hospital delivers is still the same but just costs more. The product *is* better, but probably better only in a narrow technical sense, and it is difficult to evaluate how many of these technical improvements benefit the patient.

Medicare and Medicaid played a critical role in reaching the current high level of medical technology. These federal insurance programs, introduced in 1966, created an unprecedented opportunity for physicians and hospital administrators to improve the quality of care. Fuchs argues that rather than having a major impact on health, these improvements, which included more equipment, more personnel, and more tests, may have represented the fulfillment of the hospitals' "technological imperative," and, in any case, certainly increased the cost of care. Victor Fuchs describes a case study by Professor Bernard Friedman of the treatment of breast cancer in six Boston hospitals that illustrates this concept of "technological imperative":

> In 1965, prior to the introduction of Medicare and Medicaid, about 20 percent of the cases were treated with both surgery and radiation, the other 80 percent of the cases received only one or the other treatment, at least initially. In 1967 more than 40 percent of (apparently similar) cases received initial treatment of both surgery and radiation.[13]

Friedman cannot be certain that the change in treatment was due to Medicare, since women under sixty-five also experienced changes in treatment. It may be argued that a new standard of care came into being as a result of this legislation, or that a new approach to treating breast cancer would have come about anyway, but few people would disagree that this legislation had a massive impact on hospital costs.

Berry has yet another perspective on rising costs. He explains increased hospital expenditures as the result of increased demand leading to increased prices, which in turn lead to increased net revenues employed to better the quality and extent of services, all ultimately leading to increases in the cost of hospital care over time.[14] Berry subscribes to the view that inflation in the hospital sector "has exceeded general inflation for an extended period by a significant order of magnitude" and can be explained by such characteristics as higher real incomes, population growth, a change in the population mix, and an increase in both public and private insurance coverage that has led to increased demand for hospital care. This demand, he claims, has led to higher prices, which have in turn led to an increase in net revenues. These higher revenues have been used in large part to increase both the quality and complexity of services provided with a consequent increase in the cost of hospital care over time.[15] Berry emphasizes that behavior factors are also involved, inasmuch as it is in the best interest of the trustees, the medical staff, and the administration to have the best-equipped, highest-quality hospital with the broadest services. He adds, "As profit motivated hospitals will react to an increase in demand in a way that would increase their profits, nonprofit hospitals will react to an increase in demand in a way that will increase their prestige."[16]

Regardless of the reasons for the increase in costs, it seems clear that costs have risen dramatically. While ceilings of various sorts have been imposed on hospitals, including wage and price controls and stringent reimbursement formulas, they have not done the job, and costs continue to inflate. Managerial changes seem to be a good alternative—more effective use of personnel, the establishment of a cost accounting system that prices services more realistically, and the initiation of shared services with neighboring institutions. MHSs often allow hospitals to achieve these changes, and to hire a level of management sophistication that is difficult for a small institution to justify.

Changes in Capital Financing for Hospitals

While costs have been rising in every sector of the delivery system, banks that specialize in short-term loans have generally met financing needs. If a hospital attempted to obtain funds from the capital markets, the options were quite limited and the restrictions imposed were stringent. Lenders tended to view hospitals as a real estate investment and, because they wanted to avoid the publicity of possible foreclosure, they generally gave hospitals a low loan-to-value ratio—usually less than 50 percent. Since 1966, however, when the Medicare and Medicaid legislation was enacted, patient revenues have become dependable enough for lenders to allow hospitals to increase their debt ratios. This legislation also led to an increased demand for hospital services, which led to greater a need for renovation as well as for new facilities. Health care construction costs during this period grew by 145 percent while the GNP grew by 11 percent.[17] Gradually, debt has become the predominant financing alternative, especially since levels of philanthropy have decreased sharply (see Table 2.2).

In 1977, for example, the issuance of tax-exempt bonds for financing hospitals in the United States climbed to a record $4,731,494,875 for 346 issues, exceeding the 1976 record level of $2,725,976,000 for 255 issues. These bonds accounted for 10.5 percent and 7.1 percent of the long-term municipal bond market in those years.[18]

While there is little agreement about the exact amount of future capital needs, it seems clear that needs will at least equal present-day needs. Because of the regulations imposed upon hospitals that in many states have sharply curtailed the number of new building projects by means of Certificate of Need legislation, it is possible that new investment will be more for replacement and for outpatient facilities than for the expansion of inpatient beds. Increasing reliance is likely to be placed on debt funds; some estimate that by 1981 debt will provide 80 percent of a community hospital's outlay. However, the cost of this debt is likely to increase. Today, hospitals are highly leveraged. Their debt

Table 2.2. Philanthropic and Federal Contributions to the Construction of Health Care Facilities (in Millions of Dollars and by Relative Percentage)

Year	Total Cost	Philan-thropic Contri-butions	% of Total	Federal Contri-bution (Hill–Burton Grants)	% of Total
1929	$ 207	$102	49.0	$ —	—
1935	58	10	17.0	—	—
1940	131	31	24.0	—	—
1945	139	30	22.0	—	—
1948	349	62	18.1	74	21.2
1949	679	101	14.9	75	11.1
1950	737	172	23.3	150	20.3
1955	673	177	26.3	96	14.2
1960	1,102	268	24.3	184	16.7
1961	1,174	328	27.9	184	15.6
1962	1,406	432	30.7	209	14.8
1963	1,546	455	29.4	217	14.0
1964	1,762	599	34.0	216	12.0
1965	1,837	647	34.0	217	11.8
1966	1,903	619	31.0	257	13.5
1967	1,930	650	33.6	267	13.8
1968	2,164	524	24.2	265	12.2
1969	2,500	450	17.9	n.d.	n.d.
1970	3,291	n.d.	n.d.	295	8.9
1971	3,550	n.d.	n.d.	172	4.8
1972	4,081	n.d.	n.d.	n.d.	n.d.
1973	4,145	730	17.6	46	1.1
1974	4,427	775	17.5	110	2.5
1975	4,500	705	15.6		

Sources: Social Security Administration, *Social Security Bulletin,* February 1975; American Association of Fund-Raising Counsel, Inc., "Giving U.S.A." (New York, 1975); Herbert E. Klarman, "Role of Philanthropy in Hospitals," *American Journal of Public Health* 52:8(August 1962); and C. Rufus Rorem, "Capital Financing for Hospitals" (Health and Hospital Planning Council of Southern New York, Inc., June 1968).

n.d. = no data available.

capacity is shrinking as they become increasingly risky investments, since cost containment measures are increasing the spread between cost of services and reimbursable expenses. Consequently, the industry is extremely vulnerable.

Toomey and Toomey have a slightly different, but useful, perspective on these same issues.[19] They argue convincingly that these changing modes of capital formation are influencing the capital allocation process, and see this continuing influence as an indication that the gap between the profit and nonprofit sectors is narrowing. Traditionally, the cost of capital has been a critical factor for the firm in the private sector; the firm with the lowest cost of capital had a clear competitive edge. In the not-for-profit voluntary sector of the hospital industry, capital has been accessible at a very low cost, a cost that has generally been limited to compliance with construction standards, as most hospitals benefited from Hill–Burton funds and from philanthropic donations. To make the situation even easier, no dividends were paid on that equity.

Toomey and Toomey argue that the situation has changed dramatically. Hill–Burton money now extracts dividends in terms of "a reasonable amount of charity care. In effect, the federal government is a firm investing its dollars in a hospital and exercising its rights as a stockholder by demanding dividends. The nature of the dividends happens to be humanitarian, but it is a method of investing money to develop, maintain, or prevent the deterioration of human capital."[20] Until this happened, hospital equity was free; now, the not-for-profit voluntary hospital must deal with the cost of capital as well as with the difficulty of acquiring it. Greater use of debt financing for long-term capital projects will increase the aggregate cost of hospital capital significantly. The hospital, if it is to make a realistic decision, must weigh the costs of Hill–Burton contributions or other government subsidies carrying an equity cost against financing from private sources that carries a long-term debt cost. This shift in approach is a difficult one for the hospital; to compound the problem, few hospital administrators are sophisticated money managers.

Toomey and Toomey make interesting comparisons between the private and hospital sectors that shed additional light on the financial plight of the hospital. In a private enterprise, the market and the owners or stockholders are different groups. In the case of the public community hospitals, the difficulty of obtaining philanthropic and federal dollars is forcing an increased dependence on local tax dollars, making the traditional market—the community—the same as the ownership group. These stockholders, even if they do not call themselves such, will want to exercise their ownership rights. Toomey and Toomey assert that this change represents a cost of equity to the hospital that it must take into account.

This cost of equity has an obvious financial impact on the hospital, but it also has an impact on the institution's operations. The decision to purchase an expensive piece of machinery that is likely to have a low utilization rate can no longer be made on the basis of how many physicians say they need it, but on whether it can be justified to the stockholders. These stockholders can take various forms. In the

Springvale Hospital System (see Chapter 5) they exist in the form of advisory bodies; in other hospitals they may not as yet exist at all. It seems clear, however, that community groups will take an increasingly active role in the operations of the hospital, as local monies represent a larger share of the hospital's funds.

Because of their size, which generally makes each individual unit less financially vulnerable, MHSs are in a much stronger position to obtain capital as well as to sometimes receive preferred interest rates. The St. John's Homes and Hospital Society is a good example of this; the system has a $14 million line of credit and can expand and renovate facilities where necessary. Most of the ninety-one member units would be unable to acquire the necessary capital on an individual basis.

Changes in Expectations on the Part of Both Consumers and Physicians Concerning the Role of the Hospital

The significant increase in demand for hospital services that came about after the enactment of Medicare and Medicaid has gradually led to a higher level of consumer sophistication concerning the role of the hospital. These changes have manifested themselves both in overt ways, such as a significant increase in the number and amount of malpractice suits, and in covert ways, such as the trend towards such demedicalization as "birth rooms."[21] Multihospital systems can often afford to be·more responsive to both consumers and physicians since flexibility of services is easier to attain with a larger base of assets.

It might be asked why so much attention has been placed on the hospital rather than on the many other component parts of the health system. There are indeed other providers of care, ranging from "surgicenters," which represent an attempt to perform on an outpatient basis some procedures that have traditionally been done on an inpatient basis, to long-term convalescent centers, which represent another attempt to free the hospital bed for the patient needing acute, short-term care. Nevertheless, the hospital is responsible for the greatest proportion of health costs and is indeed the focus of the American delivery system.

There is little agreement on what role the hospital should play within the delivery system—whether the hospital is the only voluntary institution capable of coordinating community health services and providing the fiscal and qualitative controls needed to create a more rational or less fragmented system, or whether the hospital is just one of many community health institutions and should not be allowed to play a central role. At this time, since the hospital does play the central role in delivering care, it is the focal point in the controversy among economists about whether increased utilization is the key factor in increased prices.

Hospitals have traditionally been able to operate with relatively little attention to the needs of consumers beyond basic "hotel" concerns. Their main concern was that of pleasing the physician, for it has been the physician who determines the census of the hospital.

During the nineteenth century, urban workers and the poor generally turned to medical charity in cases of illness—that is, to dispensaries and to hospital outpatient departments. Dispensaries were first established in England and France in the seventeenth century to provide medical advice to the needy. Gradually these dispensaries evolved into facilities where care could be given. This function was reinforced with physicians who needed medical experience, a motive that gradually led to the development of outpatient departments.[22] The first U.S. dispensary was organized in Philadelphia in 1786. In 1800 there were four dispensaries; by 1900 there were about a hundred. Although the growth of dispensaries was concentrated in the East, by 1922 some 8 million persons were receiving care.[23] There was no assumption during the early part of this century that the poor—or anyone else, for that matter—were entitled to care. As early as 1868, the *Boston Medical and Surgical Journal* commented on the needless increase in free dispensary and hospital treatment, pointing out that it was a vital injury to young physicians who had to live on the small fees obtainable from "just those middling classes of the community whom the dispensary system invites to a gratuitous treatment."[24]

Clearly conflicting interests were involved in this situation. On the one hand, physicians welcomed the teaching material, but on the other, contemporary social thought buttressed those who believed that to provide gratuitous treatment to the poor would demoralize them. This basic conflict still exists today, although significant changes have occurred on the part of both physicians and consumers as to what can reasonably be expected from the medical system.

Consumers who argue for increased outpatient care, responsive physicians and consistently high quality attention make certain assumptions about the role of the hospital, and it is not at all clear whether these assumptions are realistic.

The consumer's expectations about the role of the hospital have been altered quite drastically. Once seen as a place where one received care only as a last resort—and with a fairly poor prognosis at that, the hospital is now supposed not only to provide competent medical attention but often to coordinate family counseling, mental health activities in general, family planning, and a number of other short- and long-term therapeutic functions of which medical attention is only one. The need, says John Knowles, former Director of Massachusetts General Hospital, is "the development of comprehensive services, hospital based, extending all the expertise and the resources of the hospital out into the community health centers in conjunction with local care institutions and stimulated through federal legislation."[25] This is not to say that it is impossible for the hospital to perform all of these tasks, but it does seem quite clear that hospitals are finding it increasingly more difficult to do so, even with the best intentions.[26]

The principal problem stems from the financial obstacles discussed in the last section—a fundamental mismatch between today's needs and the hospital's ability to provide those needs. The large hospitals in urban centers are forced to handle the care of the poor who have few other resources, while at the same time serving as tertiary centers providing highly sophisticated backup for smaller hospitals, such as open heart surgery and kidney dialysis. While care of the poor never paid its own way, contributions formerly made up the difference. This is no longer true, however. In New York City, for example, where the voluntary hospitals care for more of the poor than do most urban voluntaries because New York has relatively few public hospitals, Columbia–Presbyterian reported in 1974[27] that the Vanderbilt Clinic spent $40 on each outpatient visit, charged $22, and collected whatever fraction of that $22 that it could. In effect, the larger the number of outpatients treated, the larger was the incurred deficit.

It is not only consumers who have unclear expectations about what role the hospital can and should play. Physicians play a considerably more important role since, as we have said, they are the ones who really determine utilization. Traditionally, hospitals were established in this country so that doctors would have a place to practice, as physicians found that the hospital was superior to the home or office as a place in which to care for the seriously ill. Thus, meeting the needs of the individual physicians became a primary goal for the hospital. During this period, the individual practitioner was extremely powerful. He admitted "his" patients, issued orders which were carried out without questions, and was solely responsible for the care provided.

Following the Flexner report[28] and the development of specialization, hospitals began to develop an additional goal: patient care of high quality. At first, this goal was frequently at odds with the goals of the hospital as the doctor's workshop, but quality of care eventually became the primary goal of most hospitals; it has now been institutionalized in the form of internal audits and, more recently, Professional Standards Review Organizations (PSRO). This attention to the quality of care, coupled with the availability in the hospital of better diagnostic equipment, facilities, and support staff as well as with the growth of voluntary insurance, has put tremendous pressure on the hospital. Demands are conflicting, causing problems for patients, physicians, and administration.

> On the one hand, there is an organized chorus of labor and public representatives demanding greater efficiency and less cost. On the other side the users are less vocally, but just as effectively, demanding that the hospital let the third party payers worry about costs and that the hospital concentrate on meeting the needs and the desires of the users of its services. Somewhere in between these two sides is a variety of other interests trying and succeeding in exerting special pressures on the manner in which hospitals operate.[29]

Physicians, who demand a high-quality, well-equipped, convenient place to which they can refer their patients, represent one of these interests. This pressure for convenience conflicts with health planners' demand for a more practical development of hospitals regarding optimum size and optimal use of expensive personnel and equipment. Despite these various demands, the hospital has succeeded fairly well in satisfying the different interest groups.

A number of authors have shed additional light on this question of changing expectations about the use and effectiveness of the hospital. Ivan Illich argues that improvement in health has had relatively little to do with modern medicine or with hospitals, and that, in fact, the hospital is probably the last place one wants to be. He believes that the era of the hospital as a place to treat all illnesses is coming to an end:

> The age of hospital medicine, which from rise to fall lasted no more than a century and a half, is coming to an end. Clinical measurement has been diffused throughout society. Society has become a clinic . . . the acute problems of manpower, money access, and control that beset hospitals everywhere can be interpreted as symptoms of a new crisis in the concept of disease. This is a true crisis because it admits of two opposing solutions, both of which make present hospitals obsolete. The first solution is a further sickening medicalization of health care, expanding still further the clinical control of the medical profession over the ambulatory population. The second is a critical, scientifically sound demedicalization of the concept of disease.[30]

Illich questions the use of the hospital for nontraumatic situations and argues that, in traumatic situations, its use may be warranted even less:

Intensive care is but the culmination of a public worship organized around a medical priesthood struggling against death. The willingness of the public to finance these activities expresses a desire for the nontechnical functions of medicine. Cardiac intensive care units, for example, have high visibility and no proven statistical gain for the care of the sick. They require three times the equipment and five times the staff needed for normal patient care; 12 percent of all graduate hospital nurses in the United States work in this heroic medicine. This gaudy enterprise is supported, like a liturgy of old, by the extortion of taxes, by the solicitation of gifts, and by the procurement of victims.[31]

While Illich makes some provocative arguments, which are useful because they force a questioning of the role or the usefulness of the hospital, he does not seem to take into account the many beneficial aspects of the "medicalization process." It also seems important for both consumers and physicians to retain a sense of perspective about the good that can be derived from medicine as we know it.

Superb care is available, albeit not consistently, and it can be argued that what health is and what it might be are two different things.[32] According to Fuchs:

Historians of medicine now mostly agree that it was not until well into the twentieth century that the average patient had better than a fifty–fifty chance of being helped by the average physician.

Today, at least in developed countries, the situation is markedly different. First, there is a core of medical knowledge that contributes greatly to life expectancy . . . That portion of medicine that is most dramatically effective, such as vaccines and anti-infectious drugs, is relatively simple and inexpensive to administer. But once base levels of medical sophistication, personnel, and facilities become available, additional inputs of medical care do not have much effect. In other words, the total contribution of modern medical care to life expectancy is large, but over the considerable range of variation in the quantity of medical care observed in developed countries, the marginal contribution is small.[33]

Whether we are talking about the expectation of what kind or to what extent pain is "normal," or what kind of hospital care at what cost to whom is "right," assumptions about these issues have changed as quickly as the cost of care has risen, and these changed perceptions play a major role in finding solutions for health delivery problems.

Planning Efforts as a Result
of These Problems

These problems have always existed to varying degrees, and there is not a hospital that can call itself problem-free. Planners have addressed these problems both nationally and regionally with a variety of legislation.

The word "planning" has been used in the literature both narrowly and broadly to describe such activities as cost control, problem solving, consensus formation and community decisionmaking. There appears to be extremely little consensus as to what planning is or what it is meant to accomplish in terms of the health care system. Some definitions indicate the range of thought:

Planning is the process of thinking before you act. It is reciprocally related to action, but planning itself is not action . . . I would like to add that effective planning requires that thinking be done systematically, that it is enhanced by the use of all available tools, including data; that it provide insight into the problems that must be resolved; that it is done by a number of people interacting with each other under the direction of a responsible individual; that it is done in conjunction with other organizations and individuals who have related responsibilities; that its purpose is to advise those responsible for making decisions for taking action; and that it is a continuous major function of every organization.[34]

Planning is the rational application of funds.[35]

Planning is a mechanism by which the establishment entrenches itself in such a way that would-be newcomers cannot budge them . . . Planning is a vehicle by which the establishment has feathered its own nest.[36]

Planning is not a self-justifying process; e.g., 'We pursue planning endlessly' . . . as if you did not have to justify yourself further than to say that planning is a good end in itself. And certainly, it is not.[37]

Posner implies the above definition when he describes the Vietnam approach to planning: "If you have failed in what you have done, the answer is to expand the scope of your activity."[38]

Most views of health planning agree, insofar as planning is thought to be a means of correcting for "some situation in which decentralized decision makers face inappropriate incentives. In such a situation one may attempt to change the incentives or centralize the decision process. There is no assumption a priori that either is better."[39] The question of accountability is felt by many to be the key issue in health services planning and regulation. It revolves around a basic disagreement as to where the power to make decisions should reside—in the public trust to be guaranteed by government, or in the private sector, guaranteed by free enterprise. If the government is ultimately going to be held accountable, then should it be the state or the local or the federal government, or perhaps a combination of these? This issue has never been resolved and probably can no more easily be resolved than the issue of federal versus state power or that of capacity of the individual to subordinate his interests to those of the community. While Illich would argue that the pursuit of health should be left entirely to the individual, who should be encouraged to promote his own well-being and not rely on the "medicalization" of society, it is not at all clear that a lack of federal planning would improve the fragmented health system. Robert Groose points out that one should distinguish not between a market system and a planned system, but between a planned system and a "mindless approach which lets whatever forces—political, planning, market—move ahead without the application of social conscience and community decision and without thought as to improvement of the market.[40]

The presence of the piecemeal body of planning and regulation efforts and the contradiction of laws and programs directed at the health industry reflects the very different assumptions that planners and critics make about the ability of man to subordinate personal interests to those of the community, and to whether or not power should be centralized or decentralized. Thus, it is not surprising that a wide variety of planning efforts have been initiated, each not replacing the one before it but adding to it, usually without the benefit of additional funds.

The Hill–Burton Hospital Survey and Construction Act

Health planning on a large scale is a relatively new function. Before the second World War, planning—particularly government planning—was considered vaguely Communistic and clearly un-American.[41] The Hill–Burton Hospital Survey and Construction Act of 1946 represented the first major planning effort in the medical field. It required a state-by-state survey of needs for hospital beds and established a number of other priorities, notably an emphasis on new rather than rehabilitated institutions. The implicit objective was to redistribute physicians from urban to both less urban and rural areas.

Hill–Burton was a particularly critical piece of legislation in that it encouraged a provincial attitude that already existed towards health facilities. Now every town could and was expected to have not only its own basketball team, high school, and Congregationalist church, but also its own hospital, regardless of the location and type of hospital available in the adjoining community. This approach to planning, where regionalization is viewed as a negation of personal rights, can be found today whenever any effort is made to induce communities to work together, each losing something in the process of gaining a more efficient and perhaps more effective system.[42] The effects of the Hill–Burton legislation are still evident, regardless of the legislation that superimposed on it, such as Certificate of Need (which in fact inhibits new construction, particularly in those cases where similar and probably underutilized facilities exist regionally).

It is difficult to separate planning from regulation in the health field, inasmuch as planning efforts often limit the autonomy of an organization and hence regulate its activities. Traditionally, the planning impetus came from hospital associations, who took it upon themselves to collaborate. These early planners resisted federal regulation, particularly punitive controls. In general, these early planning efforts were ineffective; hospitals were willing to collaborate but not willing to give up any form of autonomy. Gradually, planning and regulation began to have more similarities. For example, the Hill–Burton law required that hospitals give a "reasonable amount" of free care before the government would reimburse them for capital expenditures,[43] unless a waiver, based on the hospital's financial hardship, was granted. This condition was intended to address the problem of access to care for the poor, since nonpublic hospitals do not provide significant amounts of free or below-cost patient services. Although virtually all hospitals receiving Hill–Burton grants signed contractual agreements to abide by this condition, the requirement was generally ignored and unenforced.[44] Yet this kind of planning effort was quite clearly meant to have regulatory force.

Regional Medical Program

The two other major planning efforts besides Hill–Burton were also planning acts, although again they indirectly regulated the industry. The 1965 Regional Medical Program legislation (P.L. 89–239) made federal funds available specifically to achieve regional coordination of medical care delivery and to enhance the quality of care. The focus of this program was categorical, centered on cancer, heart disease, and stroke, but the program lacked focus. This was not surprising, inasmuch as its funds were limited and its purpose was "to improve the health manpower and facilities available to the nation . . . and to accomplish these ends without interfering in the patterns or the methods of financing, or patient care, or professional practice, or with the administration of hospitals."[45] This clause made it extremely difficult for substantive programs to be established to occur. In the eighteen regional medical programs studied by a team from Arthur D. Little, a large consulting firm, the only innovations and real impact on health came about in those situations where a powerful local leader co-opted the federal funds and used them for a specific purpose.

Comprehensive Health Planning Act

The Comprehensive Health Planning Act (CHP) was an enabling act designed to establish a mechanism for broad-scale health planning in all states. It was meant to give the states considerable latitude in planning based on their own needs by providing funds that were "block" grants rather than "categorical" grants—that is, funds for general rather than specific use. However, it was not clear to HEW that the states had the personnel, the skills, or the resources to evaluate their own health needs, so provisions were incorporated into the legislation to develop these capabilities in the states. The result was an extremely ambitious program whereby the states were expected to institute comprehensive health planning. Given the expansiveness of this legislation, it is hardly surprising that few states lived up to federal expectations. A survey conducted in mid–1974, seven years after the legislation became effective, revealed that only four states had established state-level plans, and that only Michigan had completed area-wide plans for each area of the state.[46] In effect, what was meant to be comprehensive health planning became subordinate to the states' health programs. In addition, the financial structure of the Comprehensive Health Planning Act was such that half of the support was to be raised locally; and the rigid requirements regarding membership on the policymaking boards discouraged local governments and traditional voluntary groups from making applications. To make matters worse, regulatory functions were quickly added to the planning responsibilities, meaning these agencies were expected to regulate the same groups in the community from which they were gaining half their support.[47] Additionally, there was a certain "more bang for the buck" philosophy in the funding of CHP agencies, whereby grants to large metropolitan areas were clearly favored on the premise that these agencies would have the largest impact on the largest number of people in the shortest length of time. While this philosophy may be pragmatic in terms of allocating scarce resources, the result, not surprisingly, was that the areas receiving less support were large, remote rural regions. Curran sums up quite well the folly of this early form of comprehensive health planning:

> . . . too many old structural legal and administrative models were utilized, too many other federal objectives were sought along with the central purpose. It was as if an engineer were asked to build a supersonic jet aircraft using only parts from old World War I gasmasks and then found that he was also supposed to make his aircraft available as a musical instrument to accompany patriotic renditions of the national anthem.[48]

Public Law 93–641

In 1975, the reorganization of the Comprehensive Health Planning program took place with the passage of Public Law 93–641, designed to remedy all the problems inherent in the first piece of legislation. It is not limited to health planning, and incorporates a new health facilities construction program, replacing Hill–Burton; it requires the states to establish certificate-of-need regulatory programs for health facilities and provides for six demonstration projects for state rate-setting programs. The key issue here is that, while the new law has considerably more scope than CHP, it does not have the additional funds required for the activities it mandates, thereby assuring that sanctions, if they are to occur at all, will be slow in coming. This is particularly true in the establishment of Health Systems Agencies (HSAs) to replace area-wide CHP bodies, which remain grossly underfunded and understaffed. HSAs are theoretically to receive a larger budget based on a per capita allotment that was not built into the earlier CHP financing, but to date, they do not have the financial capability to have a significant impact on state planning, although they do perform a myriad of statistical and administrative tasks.

Cost Control Measures

Along with these planning efforts, there have also been clearly delineated regulation efforts initiated as cost control measures. In their *Analysis of State and Regional Health Regulation,* Lewin and Associates, Inc., outlined four common cost control methods employed by both public and private third-party payers.[49]

1. Disallowing specified cost items from third-party reimbursement formulae, such as research, education related to patient care, excessive interest and depreciation costs, and bad debts.
2. Rate review: This strategy requires that changes in reimburse-

ment rates be established with the concurrence of outside agencies.

3. Capital expenditures and services (CES) controls: This approach discourages or prevents the establishment of unneeded facilities and services and deals directly with the capital formation issue, which many view as the crux of the cost containment problem.

4. Utilization Control Claims Review: This approach is meant to reduce utilization of services through such techniques as PSRO, Medicaid Utilization Review, and others.

These control measures can be characterized by their reactive nature, much like Certificate of Need legislation which now exists in twenty-five states and is based on the belief that uncontrolled growth and expansion of hospitals are largely responsible for the growing costs of hospital care. (It must be reiterated that this growth on the part of hospitals can be directly traced back to the Hill–Burton legislation discussed earlier.) Although Certificate of Need is meant to represent rational planning, it can only react to the institutions' own plans to increase facilities or services. This is done usually by stipulating a dollar amount for capital expenditures which require review.

Another method of control has been to affect what the physician does within the hospital. Many would argue that the physician's work in the hospital and, thus indirectly, the hospital's performance, has been subject to review for decades. But this review has been at best subtle and at worst criminally ineffective, with little quality standard applied to it other than that of fraud. The recent rise in malpractice legislation is one aspect of the trend towards greater accountability; the enactment of the modifications in the Social Security law in 1972 to include mandated Professional Standards Review Organizations (PSROs) provides another method of control. While at present only hospital review is mandated, it is clear that the intent is eventually to review all medical care and there is underspread controversy about the advantages or the effectiveness of this legislation.

This issue of reactive legislation is critical. Except for the early planning on the part of the hospitals themselves, which, as we have seen, did not lead to a more rationally planned health care system, most of the legislation—whether it had as its goal to plan or to regulate—has been reactive. Consequently, planning agencies, the federal authorities, and hospitals have found themselves in antagonistic positions which, in turn, has not made planning any easier.

In general, planning measures have only had limited success. Regional Medical Programs, for example, were successful in those areas where a strong individual seized the initiative and established programs that increased the scope and availability of care in certain areas, specifically heart disease, stroke, and cancer. However, the amount of money made available was negligible. Consequently, it was at best seed money and in the long run had little impact on the delivery of care.

The Comprehensive Health Planning Act made little effort to provide resources at the state level for administrative staff while at the same time proposing an ambitious plan for establishing a mechanism for broad scale health planning. CHP further assured its own demise by combining regulatory and planning functions in one agency.

Recent legislation, specifically PL 93–641, focuses on cost containment measures. Again, funds for the administration of this ambitious venture are limited; sanctions are by no means assured. The success of this legislation, if it occurs, will be largely due to the growing consumer awareness of rising costs and to subsequent community pressure on hospitals to contain costs, rather than to the legislation alone. In a similar vein, such measures as Utilization Review and PSRO will in the long run succeed in those instances where there is already a tradition of peer supervision. The observant physician is likely to become more observant; the slipshod practitioner is unlikely to be affected by such measures.

Collaboration as a Form of Planning

As these regulatory measures have increased in scope and complexity, many hospitals as well as other health care providers have felt threatened and unable to control their own operations and growth. Consequently, many health care organizations are establishing formal and informal alliances that will enable them to function with some degree of self-determination. Indeed, PL 93–641 now encourages, if not mandates, collaboration. Rather than signaling the end of financial and operational autonomy for individual institutions, collaboration is a form of active rather than reactive planning, giving those who have traditionally determined organizational goals—trustees, physicians, and administrators—some freedom to establish new relationships on the basis of goals they have themselves negotiated.

Collaboration can be considered the direct result of the problems discussed in the earlier part of this chapter, and a natural response to the planning efforts discussed in the previous section. As legislators show a greater propensity to regulate health care costs; as consumers' expectations become more sophisticated; as community representatives demand a part in the planning process; and as funds become more limited, collaboration makes more and more sense, since it allows hospitals to largely determine their own fate by working with other institutions, rather than by being controlled as a result of regulation. This is not to say that hospitals favor collaboration over autonomous behavior. It has traditionally not been in the interest of the individual institution to work with other institutions. In fact, behavior that to the planner and regulator has often seemed absurd, such as the acquisition of an extraordinarily expensive piece of machinery that is unlikely to be efficiently utilized, has to the institution in question been quite rational. Acquisition of such a gadget has meant that Board-certified physicians would be attracted to that particular department, that the community would feel positive about having a "full-facility" local hospital, and that funds would thus be easier to obtain. This goal of protecting one's self-interest has not changed; it is just attained differently in this new environment. For many institutions, collaboration—whether it be an informal alliance such as a consortium, whereby facilities and staff are shared, or a full-fledged merger, whereby a new organizational form is established—is the only reasonable action, given the environmental and financial pressures.

The number of collaborative arrangements among hospitals in the U.S. is impossible to enumerate. Collaboration can exist on an ad hoc basis, where two or more hospitals work together to attain a specific goal, or it can exist on a more permanent basis, where, for example, the institutions in question build a new facility together. The form of collaboration can range from the most informal arrangement, whereby administrators and trustees of the local hospitals conduct serious business over lunch together[50] in a private location, to a formal arrangement such as a consortium where, for example, physicians may have privileges at all hospitals in question. It is extremely difficult to judge the "success" of an arrangement, and this question of performance and performance measures will be addressed at a later point. An arrangement can be successful in the sense of saving costs for member institutions and yet be considered "unsuccessful" to staff members who feel alienated within the new arrangement. One might say that if the arrangement, continues to exist for five years or more, it has been successful.

Richard Wittrup, chief executive officer at Affiliated Hospitals Center in Boston, divides the possible relationships into four categories, while at the same time stressing that these divisions are not mutually exclusive: shared services, affiliations, mergers, and consortia.[51] He defines a shared service as "a centralized service unit serving more than one hospital and operating under hospital control or arranged for by a group of hospitals acting in consort." These can be characterized as business arrangements entered into because of operating convenience, savings in operating costs, or because the desired service cannot be obtained in another way. Typically, the arrangement is formalized in writing and each party is responsible for payment of that portion of the service consumed.

Shared services can be provided under a variety of organizational arrangements. One hospital can provide the services and sell it to the other institutions, or shared services can be organized as a cooperative venture. The critical difference between the shared service and other institutional collaborative arrangements is that member hospitals can withdraw from the arrangement at relatively low cost, and shared services are usually routine services which, albeit necessary for efficient operations, do not bear critically on a hospital's programs or its relationships with the outside world.[52]

Affiliations describe an arrangement whereby two or more hospitals are engaged in a single program, each being responsible for separate parts of this program. An example of this might be the relationship between a hospital and a neighborhood health center, where one provides in-house acute, short-term care, and the other provides the outpatient care. Affiliation usually implies that the service in question could not be provided in the same manner without the cooperation of the hospitals in question; thus, the relationships tend to be financial and political as well as purely business arrangements. The political factors become particularly important if, as so often happens, the parties in question are not equal in size and power. Affiliations can, of course, be broken, but it is considerably more difficult to renegotiate a new medical school affiliation than a new elevator maintenance contract.

Wittrup describes a merger as the consolidation of two or more corporations into one, with the remaining entity known as the surviving corporation. The critical point about merger is that the concept of cooperation technically becomes obsolete as soon as the merger is complete, inasmuch as there are no longer separate parties to cooperate. In reality, this is by no means automatic, and most mergers are fraught with political problems as the administrative structure matures.

The fourth major form of cooperation is that of a consortium, which is by far the most complicated. While merger tends to represent a reactive solution to what are usually overwhelming financial problems, consortia represent an active planning effort on the part of a group of institutions to coordinate their planning and program development. In light of what has been discussed, however, the institutions in question think that they can attain objectives more effectively by cooperating than they can by working alone. Or, as Wittrup suggests:

. . . being unable to resolve hard issues itself, a hospital can join a
consortium and put the monkey on its back. During the time that the
consortium is being formed, the hospital can say it does not want to make
decisions which ought to wait for the new entity. After the consortium is
in place, the hospital can say that it is a matter for the consortium to
decide.[53]

Familiar external pressures provide another reason for joining a consortium. Regional planning, certificate of need, and reimbursement
policies are easier to confront as a strong body than as a single institution. Inasmuch as the members of the consortium continue to work for
themselves and usually not for the good of the other members, a
successful consortium relies heavily on expert leadership to engage in
what Wittrup calls "judicious disloyalty": "What the executive must do
is to maintain the posture of steadfastly representing the interests of
the participating hospitals while quietly coaching the opposition along
lines calculated to contribute to the consortium's goals.[54] This becomes
difficult since each member may support overall goals in principle but
is likely to have its own ideas about implementation and will be
suspicious of its partners' motives.

While these categories serve as a useful schema for understanding
various collaborative forms, it must be remembered that they are not
mutually exclusive; one form can eventually lead to another and may
be, in fact, a way to test the collaboration at little cost. Too, collaborative ventures can rarely be put into a single category. Single hospitals,
or those with small branches, may make alliances with neighboring
hospitals for shared services. Or, one hospital might affiliate with
another, receive shared services from yet another, and in turn have a
management contract with a number of other hospitals.

Multiple hospital systems represent a form of affiliation whereby
two or more hospitals or other kinds of providers are under single
management. The term is used broadly, often to describe very different
kinds of collaborative forms. An MHS can contain merged hospitals or
hospitals which have a shared service arrangement with one another.
It can exist in one location or be regional or even national. The unique
characteristic of the MHS is that its member units are under the direct
operating and strategic authority of one person. This is not to imply
that the person in question is actually in charge of the institutions on a
day-to-day basis, but that if disagreement should occur about an
operating policy, the local administrator can be overruled by the chief
executive officer of the MHS.

Johnson divides multiple unit hospital systems into two categories:[55]
multiple units in several cities, and multiple units in the same locality.

In the first group, he places the Catholic orders based on an evangelistic spirit of Christianity: through healing they reach people in widely scattered communities. However, this approach is not being pursued as vigorously as it once was, perhaps because the average length of stay has fallen from 15 to 7.6 days, significantly decreasing the size of what had traditionally been a "captive audience."

The second group comprises two components: a local hospital authority, a satellite system, and a vertically integrated system on the one hand, and the single campus, diverse ownership model commonly known as the teaching hospital on the other. This effort to reduce all MHSs to two specific types does not seem particularly useful, since it is impossible to address all the possible permutations of collaboration. A better way to categorize MHSs is by whether or not they are corporate systems. The existence of the corporate form (a number of units with a corporate headquarters that may or may not have a corporate staff), means that someone is in a position to make decisions and to establish relationships among institutions. In an unincorporated confederation of units, collaboration exists in the form of consortia where decision-making is shared and where sanctions for noncompliance must come from the members themselves.

In fact, the form of the corporate arrangement, whether it is a satellite or a chain or a vertically integrated system, does not seem to be as important for understanding how a system works, or how effective it is in terms of affecting the overall delivery of care, as how the particular group of hospitals has dealt with a number of organizational and process issues which transcend the type of structure that has evolved.

NOTES

1. Senator E. Kennedy, in U.S. Congress, *Health Care Crisis in America*, Part I, Hearings before the Subcommittee on Health, 92nd Congress, First Session, February 23, 1971, page 1.
2. Materials prepared by Jonathan Brown, Ph.D. candidate in public policy at the J.F.K. School of Government, Harvard University.
3. Walter McClure, "Reducing Excess Hospital Capacity" (Minneapolis: Interstudy, Inc., 1976).
4. This issue is of particular interest since proponents of MHSs like to talk about cost savings as a result of avoiding duplication and of more effective bed utilization. While these results can occur, they are by no means assured. As R. Wittrup has said on many occasions that bigness usually implies more services, and more services tend to cost more money.
5. Note on Capital Financing for Hospitals, Harvard Business School, #4-178-225, written by D. Millikan under the supervision of Associate Professor R. E. Herzlinger.

6. Some potential patients are left out of the decision altogether because they cannot afford care. Anne Somers (*Health Care in Transition: Directions for the Future*, Hospital Research and Educational Trust, 1971, p. 21), has observed that "some 40–45 percent of the American people—the aged, children, the dependent poor and those with some significant chronic disability—are in categories requiring relatively large amounts of medical care, but with inadequate resources to purchase such care."

7. M. Feldstein and A. Taylor, "The Rapid Rise of Hospital Costs," Council on Wage and Price Stability, Executive Office of the President, January 1977.

8. Feldstein and Taylor, "The Rapid Rise."

9. In 1973 there were two scanners in use in the U.S.; in 1977 there were 760 either in use or on order for a ratio of 1:280,000. *New England Journal of Medicine*, July 28, 1977.

10. "A Radical Prescription," *Fortune*, February 1977, p. 167.

11. Ibid.

12. *Washington Report on Medicine and Health*, April 3, 1978, p. 2.

13. Victor Fuchs, *Who Shall Live? Health Economics and Social Choice* (New York: Basic Books, 1974), p. 95.

14. Ralph Berry, "Perspectives on Rate Regulation," in *Controls on Health Care, Institute of Medicine* (Washington, D.C.: National Academy of Sciences, 1974), p. 113.

15. Ibid., p. 116.

16. Ibid., p. 121.

17. Millikan and Herzlinger, Note on Capital Financing.

18. "Hospital Financing Soars to Record $4.7 Billion—a 73.6 Percent Jump in Year," *The Weekly Bond Buyer*, January 30, 1978, p. 1.

19. National Forum in Hospital and Health Affairs, *A Decade of Implementation: The Multiple Hospital Management Concept Revisited* (Duke University, 1975).

20. Toomey and Toomey, p. 14.

21. The term "birth rooms" refers to the establishment of home-like areas within a hospital where the birth process can occur in a setting that is similar to a non-structured "home" and yet where medical intervention can quickly take place.

22. William Osler, "Remarks on the Functions of an Outpatient Department," *British Medical Journal*, June 20, 1908, p. 1470.

23. Harry Moore, *American Medicine and the People's Health* (New York: D. Appleton, 1927), p. 21.

24. "Duties of Hospital Physicians and Surgeons," *Boston Medical and Surgical Journal*, 1868, 1:399, p. 30.

25. *Fortune*, January 1970, p. 15.

26. It is interesting that V.A. hospitals have traditionally operated with a "whole man" concept: the idea that each eligible veteran not only should be treated when he comes to the hospital, but that it is the system's responsibility to keep him from getting sick in the first place.

27. "Why the Nation's Hospitals May Well Go Broke," *Business Week*, October 26, 1974.

28. Abraham Flexner, *Medical Education in the United States and Canada*, a report to the Carnegie Foundation for the Advancement of Teaching, 1910.

29. Ivan Illich, *Medical Nemesis* (New York: Pantheon, 1976), p. 166.

30. Ibid.

31. Ibid.

32. In a similar vein, Illich argues that not only have expectations about health changed, but also about pain. While pain has historically played the role of a warning signal and a safeguard, today people unlearn the acceptance of suffering as

an inevitable part of their conscious coping with reality and learn to interpret every ache as an indicator of their need for padding and pampering. Traditional cultures confront pain, impairment, and death by interpreting them as challenges soliciting a response from the individual under stress; medical civilization turns them into demands made by individuals on the economy, into problems that can be managed or produced out of existence.

33. Fuchs, *Who Shall Live?*, p. 30.
34. Symond Gottlieb, in *Regulating Health Care Facilities Construction*, p. 9.
35. Joseph P. Newhouse and J. Acton, in *Regulating Health Care Facilities Construction*, p. 9.
36. Ibid., p. 44.
37. Ibid., p. 31.
38. Richard A. Posner, "Certificate of Need for Health Care Facilities Construction: A Dissenting View," in *Regulating Health Care Facilities Construction.*
39. Ibid., p. 222.
40. *Regulating Health Care Facilities Construction*, p. 41.
41. William Curran, "Present at the Creation: Health Planning and the Inevitable Reorganization," *Health Care Management Review*, Winter 1976, p. 34.
42. This trend toward collaboration is not unique in the health field; a number of post offices throughout the country have been forced to close in an effort to contain costs and provide more efficient services.
43. Toomey and Toomey refer to this as the hospital's cost of capital.
44. Recently, court actions have been brought against hospitals on behalf of the indigent; thus, the Department of Health, Education, and Welfare defined the extent of a hospital's obligation to provide free care.
45. Elliot Krause, "Health Planning as a Managerial Ideology," in *International Journal of Health Services*, 3 (1973), p. 455.
46. W. J. Curran, J. Steel, and E. W. Ober, "Government Intervention on the Increase," *Hospitals* 49:10 (May 16, 1975), pp. 57 ff.
47. W. J. Curran, "Health Planning Agencies: A Legal Crisis?" *American Journal of Public Health* 60:2 (February 1970), pp. 359–360.
48. Curran, "Present at the Creation," pp. 33 ff.
49. Lewin and Associates, Inc., *Analysis of State and Regional Health Regulation, Part I: Report of the Study* (Washington, D.C., February 1975), pp. 1–4 and 1–7.
50. National Forum in Hospital and Health Affairs, *A Decade of Implementation*, p. 6.
51. Ibid., p. 50.
52. Ibid., p. 51.
53. Ibid., p. 53.
54. Ibid., p. 55.
55. Ibid.

Chapter 3

Research Objectives
and Methodology

It is useful to think of the variety of organizational forms as occupying a spectrum (Figure 3.1):

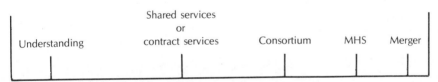

Figure 3.1. Spectrum of collaborative forms.

Movement along this spectrum is a function of the level of autonomy retained by individual institutions and of the need for interdependence. If two or more institutions have an understanding that, for example, long-range plans will be made jointly, the level of interdependence in other areas such as patient care services need not be significant. If, on the other hand, two or more institutions have established a consortium, then in all likelihood a variety of decisions will be made jointly, necessitating considerable interdependence.

While this typology of collaboration allows the researcher and the administrator to put the MHS in perspective, it does not tell us how these systems develop. This book will attempt to fill this gap by studying the developmental patterns of a sample of MHSs in order to explain the similarities and differences that characterize their evolution.

Preliminary research on different collaborative modes suggests four questions:

Is there a relationship between the system's age and its organizational effectiveness? The most extensive study[1] on this suggests that the age of the system is correlated with its ability to cope with its environment; in other words, an older system is more likely to have an effective organizational process and is able to perform tasks and achieve goals better than a younger system.

Are there environmental variables which are relevant to all MHSs regardless of their developmental stage? Each system operates in a unique environment that exerts a variety of pressures. While these pressures constantly change, research suggests that the characteristics of the environment can be categorized in such a way that the variables described could be of use to both researchers and administrators.

Can system responses be characterized in such a way that they are related to environmental demands, and do these responses occur in a certain pattern as the system develops? While each system appears to face a unique set of constraints, it seems clear that a variety of activities are undertaken that are similar regardless of the environment. For example, systems usually establish a corporate staff, make some effort to work with regulatory agencies, and develop sources of dependable revenues.

What is the relationship between the system's leader, its chief executive officer, and the development of the system? In all the systems studied either for this book or in previous work, it appears necessary for someone to effectively orchestrate the relationships between the system's headquarters and the outlying units, and to decide on what tasks are most likely to insure that the system achieve its objectives. Effective orchestration demands different roles at different times.

Each of these questions suggests a particularly relevant body of literature (see Chapter 4). For example, the first question can best be tested by first examining available work on multihospital systems. The second question suggests the literature on stages of development, the third suggests the literature on adaptation, and the fourth the literature on leadership. Figure 3.2 graphically describes the relationship between the research questions and the literature review.

Previous Research	Research Questions	Literature Review
	Is there a relationship between a system's age and its organizational effectiveness? ⟶	Literature on MHS
Hospital mergers	Are there environmental variables relevant to all MHSs? ⟶	Literature on growth and evolution of organizations
Interviews with CEOs	Are system responses related to environmental demands, and do they change over time? ⟶	Literature on organizational adaptability
	What is the relationship between the CEO and the development of each system? ⟶	Literature on leadership

Figure 3.2. Research questions.

METHODOLOGY

Available work on multihospital systems is largely descriptive; most of it makes little effort to be analytical, and often consists of a case study on one emerging organization or on the benefits of a concept such as shared services. Consequently, I have taken a clinical approach, where I established a relationship with the CEO and that permitted additional data gathering as the research progressed.

This clinical method is fraught with problems. It is harder to generalize findings from a small number of sites and it is impossible to know what one has missed by not having studied a far greater number of sites. Yet the potential depth of material is so much greater than what can be obtained from a statistical study that the risks and problems of a clinical approach seemed warranted. I felt that output from this kind of research, where managers themselves established the hypotheses, would yield the most persuasive data for other managers, who could then improve their ability to diagnose their own organizations and thus write their own prescriptions for effective change.

Methodological Issues

The decision to explore the development of the MHS led to a number of methodological issues, which included which variables to study, the time horizon, and the site selection for the study.

Variables

I chose the variables to be included according to the environmental issues relevant for each system, and the way the system acted in response to these demands; that is, the tasks or activities that it chose, and the characteristics, both personal and professional, of the chief executive officer.

The importance of one variable became evident as it was repeated by the various CEOs, suggested by the frequency and intensity of their responses.

Open-ended interviews were conducted with leaders of seven multihospital systems. The following areas were covered in the two-hour interviews:

the CEO's background
the history of the multihospital system he headed
the tasks the CEO had addressed, and which ones he thought were
    most important at the time of the interview
what environmental issues he thought the system had to consider
how he differentiated his job from those of his staff members

Considerable data was obtained during the course of these interviews and a large number of variables were included, inasmuch as little effort was made to structure the thoughts of the CEO beyond the broad categories defined above. While I did have the four major questions that I wanted to explore at the back of my mind, I wanted to understand how each multihospital system had developed and what the relationship was between the structure of the system and the tasks undertaken by the CEO. Each interview, in fact, led me to further definition and additional questions. The process was much like a puzzle. With each interview I "found" new pieces that were sometimes discarded but that sometimes provided critical linkages. These new pieces were then included in subsequent interviews.

Time Horizon

From the outset, it was clear that a longitudinal study, whereby an organization could be explored over a considerable length of time as it considered merger or affiliation and proceeded along the chosen route, would have been advisable. However, preliminary investigation suggested that the multihospital system is a delicate organizational form that does not lend itself to careful inspection until the participating members have clearly defined their roles and expectations. Unlike mergers and other forms of affiliation in the private sector, where the legal commitment to combine resources does not occur until decisions have been made concerning such difficult issues as redundancy of personnel and reporting relationships, hospitals involved in mergers and other forms of affiliation delay any solution to these issues until after they decide to merge. As a result, access to the ongoing process is usually impossible to obtain.

This critical problem dictates a study of established multihospital systems at one point in time, when organizational dynamics can be dissected and when historical perspective can be obtained by appropriate questioning. There are of course problems in studying events that have already occurred. One must trust the memory of the CEO for an accurate history of the organization, unless one can interview everyone who played a part in the collaboration. The history of most multihospital systems, however, has generally been short enough that accuracy is fairly easy to establish.

Then, to assess a system's leadership, I had to choose systems that were not in the process of radical change, and that had not recently undergone change. I thus decided to choose sites that had clearly become multihospital systems, but that had done so long enough before the interview date for the new arrangement to be functioning smoothly, but not so long ago that historical accuracy was impossible to obtain.[2]

Site Selection and Respondents

After some consideration, I decided to study some of the country's major corporate multihospital systems. My preliminary investigation strongly suggested that, among more than 400 systems of various sizes and types,[3] there existed a group of systems that had been in existence long enough to be stable, to have achieved a national reputation, and to have a leader who had been the prime mover or who had at least been present through most of the creation. I verified my theory in a number of ways:

I asked established leaders in hospital administration for the names of stable systems all of whose institutions were directed by a single leader.

During each interview, I asked the CEO what systems he would add to the list.

It soon became evident that there existed a "first cut" of hospital systems, followed by a large number of emerging systems throughout the country that I did not include in the study. I tried to include all of these major systems rather than choosing a sample, on the premise that the number of such systems was small enough to study. Letters were sent to all of the sites and, while all the CEOs in question showed interest in taking part in the study, their hectic schedules led to a number of broken appointments. The final number included in the study was seven of nine potential sites. The location of these sites led to some difficult decisions about whom to talk to and how long to spend on site.

It seemed wise to concentrate on the CEO in this exploratory work. While there is usually a large gap in experience and span of control between the CEO and his assistants, making it useful to obtain collaborative data from a number of other perspectives, it would have been difficult to do so and at the same time study all selected sites. Time and costs also made it extremely difficult to spend significant time in each site.

In addition, problems at lower levels of the organization can more easily be programmed; rules and regulations can be devised for their solution. As Selznick says, "At these lower levels we may expect to find effective use of rather simple devices for increasing efficiency and control[;] it is here that scientific techniques of observation and experiment are likely to be most advanced and most successful."[4] At higher levels, however, problems tend to "be more resistant to the ordinary approach of management experts."[5] The metaphor of the "smooth-running machine" becomes less applicable; thus it is at this level that administration becomes truly discretionary, and its study most desirable.

I also had to address the question of studying "failed" versus "successful" sites. While it did initially seem advisable to obtain data about failures as well as successes, I decided not to do so for two reasons:

It is extremely difficult to pinpoint a "failure." Does a hospital group where the relationship has remained at the "informal contract" level rather than having progressed to "total merger" or to a consortium mean that the relationship has failed? Exploratory research suggests that it has not. While some hospitals do seem to first "test the water" and move fairly rapidly from one kind of relationship to another, other hospitals appear perfectly comfortable with extremely slow movement along the same continuum.

When a situation has clearly failed, radical changes are usually being made, making information extremely difficult to obtain.

A number of other methodological issues had to be addressed. I considered many alternative approaches in developing a conceptual model that would contribute to an understanding of development in a multihospital system:

A study of a sample of institutions in each of a number of organizational forms ranging from shared services to mergers.
A study of multihospital systems over time, which would include each stage of development, concentrating on the tasks the leader must sequentially address.
A study of those multihospital systems that fit into certain categories.

I decided to exclude all organizational forms with the multiple leadership, such as consortia. While understanding interinstitutional cooperation is extremely relevant to the health delivery system, it seemed outside the scope of this study to include organizations that were working together on a purely voluntary basis. Thus, only corporate MHSs where a clearly defined leader existed were included. Additionally, I included only those systems that had been in existence for at least five years, in an effort to insure structural organizational stability.[6]

Finally, those systems that were Church-dominated or totally university controlled were excluded on the premise that their operating philosophy would be significantly different from the other systems'. The sites finally chosen were[7]:

Mid-Atlantic Regional Hospitals
Hillcrest Community Hospitals
Springvale Hospital System
Western Affiliated Hospital Society
St. John's Hospitals and Homes Society
Sun State Health Service
The Metropolitan Medical Center

The Interview Process

Every attempt was made to make the interviews as unstructured as possible while at the same time obtaining data in specific areas (see p. 38). Initially, I decided to tape the interviews, but the amount of data generated and the cost of transcribing the tapes did not seem to warrant this step. I thus tried to obtain as much information as possible about each site to avoid repeating factual data that could be obtained elsewhere, and to take notes which were then dictated at the end of each interview. This approach seemed particularly useful, inasmuch as the same people could be contacted for additional data based on the information obtained as the interviews progressed.

Too, a certain amount of spontaneity was lost by taping the interviews, particularly in one site where the CEO was especially reticent due to a previous problem with unfortunate press coverage. In all instances, CEOs were assured that the interviews were to be confidential. Much to my surprise, in three of the sites, information was given to me that could have negatively affected the operations of the system. Interviews lasted approximately two to three hours. Although I would have preferred to move from one site to another, allowing a cross-fertilization of ideas between sites, this was made impossible by the location of the seven sites. In fact, by the third or fourth interview there were a number of questions that I wished I could have gone back and asked the first respondents and I sometimes did this if the necessary information was specific enough to obtain via telephone. This methodological approach seems appropriate in that the questions asked were exploratory. There exist no models in the literature purporting to describe or explain the relationship between tasks, and the environment of health institutions within a dynamic framework. A later phase of this research could usefully apply the findings to a broad sample of multi-institutional systems in differing stages of development.

NOTES

1. For a review of this study by the AHA, please see Chapter 4.
2. This problem of when to study the systems was a particularly difficult one to solve. It was virtually impossible to have a useful discussion with the CEO if the organization was in the midst of a critical change; this hypothesis was confirmed in Detroit with an emerging consortium and again in Springfield, Mass., as three hospitals were forming a system. It can, of course, be argued that the problem was a lack of rapport between the interviewer and the interviewee, but it seems much more likely that the problem was the CEO's fear of saying anything that could jeopardize a very fragile situation.
3. M. Brown and H. Lewis, *Hospital Management Systems: Multi-Unit Organization and Delivery of Health Care* (Germantown, Md.: Aspen Systems Corporation, 1976).
4. Philip Selznick, *Leadership in Administration* (New York: Harper & Row, 1957), p. 3.
5. Ibid.
6. This is not to imply that the sites in question were not changing, for they were. In fact, it seems clear that to be effective, change is critical. But adaptive change is different from a total structural alteration.
7. The names of these systems and their CEOs have been fictionalized.

Chapter 4

Multihospital Systems: A Conceptual Framework

INTRODUCTION

In the previous chapters the phenomenon of the MHS has been explored with particular emphasis on those characteristics of the health system that led to significant alterations in the delivery of care.

The field of organizational behavior provides a rich theoretical foundation within which the development of the MHS can be viewed. In addition, some work has been done on MHSs themselves and, while this research has been descriptive rather than analytical, it is important to review it in order to place the MHS within a conceptual framework.

In Chapter 3, four research questions were asked. Each of these questions suggests a particular research area to be reviewed. The first section will discuss the work that has been done on MHSs, the second will discuss the research on the growth and evolution of organizations, the third will explore the area of organizational adaptation, and the fourth will concentrate on the literature concerning leadership.

43

THE LITERATURE ON MULTIHOSPITAL SYSTEMS

There is considerable data available on multihospital systems. Much of it, however, is statistical and is far more concerned with the effectiveness of such systems than with their development.[1]

Rutstein[2] has described this growth of systems as a partial reaction to the haphazard state of medical care characterized by a lack of coordination among hospitals. He stated that many American hospitals foolishly attempt to staff and equip themselves with over-specialized service in situations where this kind of investment cannot be justified. Rutstein foresaw that the multiple-unit organization would offer the specialist the large patient base necessary to keep his skills at peak efficiency, and concluded that the medical system had to be built around regional medical service areas centered upon large teaching hospitals affiliated with medical schools. Some multiple-unit health organizations may already function as regional services similar to Rutstein's model. In any case, there are many forms of multiple-unit organizations that can be characterized in a number of different ways.

Montague Brown, who has done considerable work classifying these systems, concludes that distinctions are becoming diffuse[3] and that the major distinctions remaining between hospitals are bed size, teaching or nonteaching, and whether in fact the hospital is part of a system. A major report published by the AHA in 1974 concludes that:

> . . . each hospital is an element of a larger environmental system from which it received its resources, a charter for its operations, and guidance or control. The key to the definition of a multiple unit health care delivery organization is *how the hospital (or individual unit)* is controlled or managed by the larger environmental system from which it draws its resources. The most important question appears to be the degree to which direct control and management responsibility emanates from a larger body or organization which *exerts decision making influence over more than one hospital or other health care delivery unit.*[4]

The AHA (Doody, 1974) defined multihospital systems as having two or more hospitals with legal incorporation and a common board with accountability, or two or more hospitals in a chain with a board to determine overall direction and provide some central direction and administrative service, or a major affiliation agreement or management contract, or lease with responsibility for central policy with or without the legal incorporation, or a common board. The key issue again here is how the decisionmaking powers of the governing authority are legitimized for the provision of services. The first method is through ownership and the second is through managerial control. If ownership responsibilities, management responsibilities, or both are assumed for more than one hospital or unit, a multiple unit, or system, has been developed.

Although little systematic attention has been paid to MHSs, a substantial amount of literature exists on the various aspects of reorganization including decisionmaking, goal setting, and coordination.

A survey of the literature reveals articles that are mostly descriptive and often based on a single case study. A major report by the AHA purports to divide original growth into two categories, "external"—whereby management and coordination of existing hospitals are subsumed under one organizational structure—and "internal," where new facilities are added to an already existing structure. This division seems somewhat arbitrary, inasmuch as most MHSs experience both kinds of growth making it difficult to say which processes fall into which division. It seems more useful to think in terms of a spectrum of activity.

There are a number of mechanisms for bringing hospitals into closer working relationships with one another. Merger tends to receive considerably more attention than the other mechanisms although it represents a relatively small number of processes. The most common type of MHS arrangement today is a system owned and operated by a religious organization; the second most common is the investor owned chain, and the third is a system consisting of merged or consolidated not-for-profit hospitals. Other mechanisms for increasing interinstitutional relationships are political ties, such as state, county, and city hospital "systems" and hospital "districts" and managerial ties, such as affiliation agreements and management contracts.

Starkweather noted in 1971 that little is known about the overall merger process or its outcome. He described health facilities in terms of static dimensions including organizational patterns, legal bonds, nature of combined services, stages and forms of production, geography or population served, facility location and organizational impact. He viewed these organizational combinations as a process having five stages with a set of economic and social conditions supportive of a future merger and ending with a formal contract between the organizations.

This typology is at best descriptive of certain merger situations and does not deal at all with the large number of affiliative agreements that are not mergers. It also does not address how the organization moves from one stage to the other or the role of management in facilitating or constraining this movement.

As to quantitative data about the precise number of hospitals that are part of a system, the most reliable data is obtained by the AHA, which compiles data according to the nine census divisions. As of 1977, there were approximately 400 systems. Of 6700 hospitals, 2300 were reported to be part of a large formal system; most of the hospitals were in the 100- to 199-bed category. (In 1968, 200 out of 7000 hospitals were in a system.) The largest number of units in a system were in Alaska, California, Hawaii, Oregon, and Washington. The smallest number of systems hospitals were located in Connecticut, Maine, New Hampshire, Rhode Island, and Vermont. The community hospital systems ranged from many systems of only two hospitals operated under a single management to 90 health care providers located in 14 states operated under a central management. Of the total 926,000 community hospital beds available in 1975, 293,000—32 percent—could be placed in the system category.[5]

THE GROWTH AND DEVELOPMENT OF ORGANIZATIONS

Most of the research in this area has been done and continues to be done on corporations in the private sector. While a comparison of the MHS and the comparable multidivisional firm is outside the scope of this book, it is useful to examine the models that have been developed in the for-profit sector in order to shed additional light on the relationship of MHSs to the environments in which they operate.

In general, models of corporate development have subdivided the history of an institution into segments or stages. Rostow[6] proposed that each stage occurs in a characteristic sequence and that these regularities stem from the managerial requirements of a similar set of activities rather than from size or "age" per se.

Through the study of the development of some seventy large American corporations, Alfred Chandler[7] found certain uniformities that appear to occur in sequence as a company develops. While it is difficult to justify that certain activities are bound to occur at a given point in time and not at another, it does seem useful to view an organization as requiring different management skills at an early stage in its development because it is in fact performing different functions than it would be at a later point. A simple unit (Stage 1) organization, for example, is:

unlikely to require specialization among its subunits because subunits are often not clearly defined.

likely to have an unsystematic and paternalistic system of rewards and punishments. The measures of performance are likely to be assessed by personal contact using subjective criteria.

On the other hand, a multiunit organization (Stage 3) is:

likely to have a significant specialization among units, each of which may in fact deal directly with one or more markets.

likely to measure performance by market criteria such as return on investment. Its reward and punishment structure is likely to be systematic, with a strong impersonal element.[8]

The MHS seems to fall in between the "single unit" (Stage 1) and the "multiunit" (Stage 3) firm. Its subunits seldom have the power to act independently in the marketplace; hence the system acts as though it were one company.

In addition to the stages models which propose different developmental patterns as a function of whether a corporation is a single unit or a multiunit, other models add a strategic component. Two companies might for example both be multiunit corporations (Stage 3) and yet embark upon very different activities because they have different strategies.

These models, while clearly inexact, are useful for facilitating comparison between, let us say, a Stage 3 Swedish steel maker with a Stage 3 American manufacturer of sewing machines, or between two competitors in the same industry. From such a comparative analysis one can begin to draw some conclusions about how different companies exploit a similar environment. Observed differences in strategy can be traced to a number of factors, among them:

different company endowments in skills and resources
differences in perception of opportunity
differing abilities to conceptualize a sequence of advantageous moves for exploiting perceived opportunities

In his recent book,[9] Chandler carries the idea of corporate growth models and strategy one step further by proposing a different managerial emphasis in each stage.

Greiner[10] adds a different perspective by proposing that each period of development is characterized by stages of evolution and then revolution necessitating a change in strategy. The author maintains that growing organizations move through five distinguishable phases of development, each of which contains a relatively calm period of growth that ends with a management crisis. Greiner feels that it is the job of the manager to turn organizational crisis into opportunities for future growth.

These models of corporate growth provide an interesting, albeit crude, framework in which to view multihospital systems. They do propose that assessment of environmental factors and changes in these conditions are a critical task for a growing corporation and that strategic decisions must be made as a consequence of this assessment. This suggests the ability of the organization to adapt in order to survive.

ORGANIZATIONAL ADAPTATION

The concept of organizational adaptation is especially important in that multihospital systems appear to have been established as a response to rapidly changing external demands that made it difficult for traditionally autonomous institutions to provide care. This response is the focus of this book. Although the question of how organizations adapt has been given little attention in the literature, contributions have been made which at least serve as a starting point.[11]

The literature on adaptation is found principally in a context related to biological or natural systems rather than social systems. In addition, it has usually been applied to profitseeking organizations rather than to public agencies or to the health sector.

The literature on cybernetics was useful in developing the notion of the multihospital system as a dynamic organism operating in a particular ecological niche. Perhaps the most useful model within the cybernetic framework was that of W. Ross Ashby.[12] The model he developed postulates that the organization develops responses to environmental stimuli, which he calls the parameters. As the essential variables exceed a predetermined limit, a new organizational response must be developed. Without this ability to sense the need for change, the organization will no longer be viable.[13]

In the health sector, environmental stimuli have been limited; consequently, little response has been needed on the part of the organization. Perhaps as a result of this, the hospital has not learned how to respond quickly and effectively. The tools do not exist because the need for utilizing them has not existed. As long as inefficient but effective care could be provided it made little sense to develop tools that would lead to more efficient care at the same level of quality.

Ashby's model, although principally concerned with natural and mechanical systems, is useful in that it presents the organization as having to go through a learning process of trial and error. It does not, however, attempt to address how it best organizes itself so that the appropriate response can be made to environmental stimuli, or how it is able to distinguish among the myriad stimuli that bombard it, only some of which are relevant.

The literature of cybernetic medicine is also relevant. Harvey[14] presents the law of requisite variety, which he feels is central to the understanding of how large systems function. This law states that in a regulator, only more variety or complexity can overcome more variety or complexity in the disturbance. It would follow, then, that in order for an organization to effectively deal with an increasingly complex environment, it would need to become more complex itself.

Research in the field of biology has emphasized the dependency of living things upon their environment, and, in fact, research in the life sciences during the past decade—particularly into pollution and its effects on the environment—has brought to light the interdependence of living systems. This notion of living things as open systems is useful; it emphasizes the fact that an organism obtains necessary elements from outside itself, processes these elements, and produces new elements. Additionally, the organism obtains information that enables it to change course and protect itself in such a way that it can continue to exist.

Actually, these ideas are not new. Roots of this "system movement" can be traced back through the literature. In 1938, for example, Chester Barnard, in *Functions of the Executive,* built an analysis around the organization as a system, beginning with his definition of an organization as a "system of consciously coordinated activities or forces of two or more persons"[15] and stressing the need to think about an organization as a whole. He saw the component parts of the organization as interdependent variables and saw the need for subsystems appropriate to this interdependency.

These ideas give us a set of concepts and working hypotheses dealing with the basic similarities existing in all systems. Looking at an organization rather than an organism with this model in mind can be quite useful and, if one does not strain the metaphor too much, the framework can help us understand the ways in which organizations work and do not work. Katz and Kahn use this framework extensively, and yet freely admit the inadequacies of the metaphor:

> The communications network of social organism bears only a distant and figurative resemblance to the physical structures, such as the circulatory and nervous systems, by which the subparts of the biological organism are integrated. Too often such loose metaphors have prevented the sociologist or even the biologist . . . from grasping the essential differences between organism and society.[16]

For one thing, the bonds which hold a social system together are considerably more tenuous than those which hold a physical system together. While an organism generally has a clearly defined objective and exists in such a way as to achieve this objective, manmade systems may have a multitude of objectives and, in fact, may change objectives during the course of their life. A moth is likely to remain a moth. Through the long process of evolution it might change, in a smoggy region, from a light moth to a slightly darker one in order to avoid detection, but it has no more power over this process than the doorbell has power not to chime if the proper connection is made. Westinghouse can switch from manufacturing refrigerators to manufacturing teaching machines. The change is not easy; it involves serious resource allocation decisions, but it *can* be made. In a physical system, the component parts themselves provide constancy; in a contrived system—an organization—the relationships of items rather than the items themselves provide constancy. Similarly, biological systems have a predictable growth curve, while contrived systems do not. Assuming normal functions, for example, a tadpole will become a frog. An organization, however, may go through periods of specifiable growth and crisis, but it may also take totally unpredictable steps, still survive, and in fact, thrive.

Just as the biological system has innumerable control mechanisms which serve to maintain it, allow it to grow, and to change, so the contrived system—the organization—also has control mechanisms. As the temperature drops, the human body reacts in a number of ways to preserve its internal temperature. As the supply of a critical raw material disappears, a company will take steps to deal with the potentially disastrous situation. It may try to replace the raw material with another one; it may co-opt the raw material (that is, buy the source itself); or it may choose to go out of business. The difference is, of course, that a given stimulus, such as a drop in temperature, *will* lead to a predictable effect in the human body, while the disappearance of a necessary raw material *may* lead to a large number of outcomes, none of which can be predicted with certainty. Mouzelis describes this kind of control mechanism as a selfsteering mechanism involved in organizational decisions.[17] The system, according to him, is made up of a detector, a censor or governor, a selector, and an effector.

Thus, we see that the metaphor that describes an organization in the terms used to describe a biological system has its limits, yet remains quite useful as a way of exploring organizations. It also becomes apparent that understanding a biological system, even a simple one, is a difficult and not yet attained feat. The challenge lies in discovering the mechanisms by which events occur: given a certain drug, why is a clinical remission seen? In studying organizations, however, the challenge lies in understanding patterns of behavior which form a set of circumstances that are *likely* to occur. Bales's[18] research, for example, tells us that in certain situations a task leader is likely to be more effective than a socio-emotional leader, but this predictive model is contingent upon a number of conditions being met.

The question, then, is how these ideas can be used in a discussion of health systems, and, more specifically, how organizations establish subunits that can effectively respond to environmental stimuli and internal stress.

Katz and Kahn see five types of subsystems that describe organizational functioning: productive subsystems, concerned with the work that gets done; supportive subsystems, which concern themselves with procurement, disposal and institutional relations; maintenance subsystems which arrange roles for interrelated performance and tie people into the system; adaptive subsystems, which are concerned with organizational change; and managerial subsystems, which are responsible for the direction and control of the various other subsystems and activities of the organization.

There is nothing in the productive, supportive, and maintenance systems to insure organizational survival in a changing environment, and it seems clear that environments *do* change.

Examples of this change are rampant; any large university provides a good example. In the past decade recruitment policies, placement policies, and curricula have all been significantly altered; these changes were largely due to adaptive mechanisms within the institution that alert it to changes in the environment that are likely to affect it. In an educational system this process is somewhat easier to accomplish than in a company, because graduates become feedback mechanisms, as do prospective applicants and professors who often consult in the very organizations likely to hire graduates.

Nonetheless, most organizational functions face inward; they are concerned with the ongoing activities of the organization rather than the activities that it might undertake. The risks of this concentration on what *is* as opposed to what *might be* are proportional to the rate of change in the environment that affects, or is likely to affect, the organization. As a result of this risk, there are formal and informal structures within most organizations to address these possible changes. These structures comprise the adaptive subsystems of the organization and may be called a wide variety of names, such as Research and Development, New Product Development, Corporate Planning, or Long Range Planning. If these adaptive subsystems did not exist, then, in all likelihood, boundaries would continue to change and the environment would continue to affect the organization in new challenging ways. However, without the capabilities to sense these changes and to react to them, the organization would continue allocating its total energies to a continuation of the status quo and perhaps find itself in serious trouble when environmental changes became so obvious that everyday operations were affected.

In the hospital, for example, consumerism as a movement of increasing force and importance has traditionally been ignored, since hospitals have tended to pay little attention to their adaptive function. As a result, a number of institutions have (much to their surprise) found themselves as a target of abuse for people who expect adequate, reasonably priced outpatient care and are incensed to find that their community hospital will not provide it. An interesting aspect of the subsystems within an organization is that they are at odds with one another—there are limited resources both in terms of staff and monies, and it is difficult to allocate these resources to an activity which is potentially important but difficult to define and justify (such as environmental scanning) when management has traditionally abided by a crisis management philosophy. This has been particularly true for hospitals where management capability has been scarce. In between the chief executive officer and the department heads (who often do not have fiscal responsibility) there has been a paucity of available and skilled people. This scarcity has made it even more difficult to appoint someone to "work with the community," "get to know the regulatory people," or "evaluate the potential effects of upcoming legislation"—all critical boundary-scanning functions.

It seems useful at this point to discuss Thompson's[19] contribution to the area of organizational adaptation. He notes that the innate tendency of an organization is to remain closed rather than open, in order to operate with what it assumes to be complete certainty. This has particularly been true of hospitals that have operated autonomously rather than as part of a system. Decisions have traditionally been made with regard only to immediate perceived needs, and often only as those needs were perceived by an individual physician. One hospital will purchase a cobalt unit, which is likely to be operated so far under capacity that a similar decision would seldom be made in a manufacturing firm. The decision will disregard not only the number of patients per year who are likely to need this facility and alternative uses for the money, but also that another hospital serving the same patient population has recently purchased the same unit, which is already operating far under capacity. As inefficient as this process might seem to the onlooker, it is quite efficient from the hospital's point of view. The funds are available for the cobalt unit, and its presence would attract a first-rate radiologist, which would appeal to the community spirit and to the Chamber of Commerce, thus allowing it to raise funds more easily for the construction of a new maternity wing, which would, in turn, also operate at a loss. Were these arguments to be pointed out to the administrator or to the physician who suggested the purchase in the first place, the argument would be made that to save just one life by means of this purchase would override all cost and other practical considerations. Thus, remaining a closed system can be a rational alternative for an institution that sees no benefit in changing its decisionmaking mechanisms.

In point of fact, the American Medical Association has devoted the past fifty years to maintaining a closed system by opposing any measures which would change health care from fee-for-service to a prepaid system. This opposition has included not only health insurance of any sort but also all forms of compulsory inoculation. Their reason for this stance was generally that such changes would constitute "bureaucratic interference with the sacred rights of the American home"[20] and would tend to promote communism.

A number of writers besides Thompson have described this organizational proclivity to remain closed. Weber, for example, saw the modern organization to be similar to the modern machine—unencumbered by whim and run by experts, all working to achieve a specific goal which could be defined and which was static.

If we assume at least a relatively open organization that attempts to obtain and process information, it becomes critical to consider Thompson's concept of boundaries to describe the interface between the organization and the environment. Most modern organizations must consider so many variables in any decision that decisionmakers consciously choose to ignore a certain number, especially those which are highly uncertain. A hospital, for example, will be very much affected by National Health Insurance. The chance of comprehensive insurance of this sort occurring in the near future is good, yet in most decisions the probable effects of such a change, albeit overwhelming, cannot be incorporated into the decision process. Thus, this variable tends to be ignored.

The result of this level of uncertainty in the environment, with which the organization must constantly contend, is to make decisions in what Thompson calls bounded rationality. Using the Simon-Cyert-March[21] idea of "satisficing" rather than "maximizing," one might say that in solving problems, the organization does not attempt to include all possible variables (maximizing) but instead attempts to include the relevant ones which can be made tangible and concrete (satisficing). Additionally, an organization operates *as if* no major changes are likely to occur in the present term or in the immediate future, in effect buffering itself, to use Thompson's term—protecting itself from environmental changes. To use the example of National Health Insurance (NHI) again, the hospital plans its growth and staffs accordingly, as if NHI were not going to occur, in order to buffer its principal activities from what might be overwhelming changes which would force it to reevaluate the number of beds it has and the number of personnel in attendance.

Just as a major piece of legislation such as NHI might force a hospital to change in a number of ways, radical fluctuations in its census might also induce change. When one considers such concepts as resource allocation and organizational slack, it seems clear that staffing patterns in hospitals are not closely correlated with census variations. Yet effective reduction of the slack in most general hospitals would be extremely difficult to accomplish, and there appears to be little incentive built into the system to work on the problem in the first place. Instead, staffing patterns are smoothed out in such a way that there are sometimes too many nurses in attendance in obstetrics (where variations are especially marked) and sometimes too few, but usually at least enough to deliver adequate care. Yet most hospitals are well aware of census variations and they become more adaptive by learning from a previous set of experiences and adjusting operations accordingly.

It seems clear that the process we are discussing as adaptation refers to an area which has received considerably more attention as "learning." The ability of a species to learn improves its chances of survival by giving it options. Hart[22] explores this at length, using the terms "learning" and "adaptability" quite interchangeably. He discusses early man, emphasizing that climate changes were the greatest motivators to learning. As fluctuations from colder to hotter and back again enormously affected climates, as well as sea level and topography, those who did not move as climates changed probably perished. For those who did adapt by moving to another location and changing their habits, surviving even briefly required new skills. Hart believes that a species only learns when more is demanded of it. If food is plentiful, for example, the organism does not need to change its habits or to adapt. If food becomes scarce, however, it must be searched for, making brain requirements rise. If food needs to be stored in order to span a projected shortage, requirements again rise. If the food supply can be invaded by smaller organisms and thus must be protected, requirements again rise. Each of these steps forces the organism to learn from the previous step so that it might adapt to a changing environment.

Thompson refers to the process by which organizations learn as "scanning." Organizations study their environment, study their past experience interfacing with this environment, and sometimes change themselves in such a way that they can adapt to relevant changes before they are forced to react by these same changes. Earlier I mentioned adequate outpatient services as a change in public expectations about hospitals. The institution that sees this change coming and initiates a home-care program, or a well-baby clinic located in a community center, or a responsive emergency room staff that understands the needs of its audience, has scanned the environment and adapted to it. It has understood that its boundaries were no longer delineated by its four walls and that, as its boundaries changed, it too had to change or perhaps be forced to change in ways it might not have chosen had it had time to choose and act accordingly.

Both the maintenance and the adaptive subsystems tend to move toward organizational growth. The maintenance subsystem attempts to maintain a steady state of equilibrium by the use of procedures, standards, and other ways of institutionalization. It is by nature conservative. The adaptive subsystem attempts to control the outside world by reacting to external pressures in such a way that the organization can change. Both systems attempt to reduce uncertainty and to make the environment more predictable. It would appear that, as the organization becomes more complex, more differentiated, it would need more formal adaptive systems that could eventually be institutionalized. Are there "adaptors" within organizations just as there are "integrators" serving a linking pin function—individuals who pay special attention to slight changes in stress that might be harmful if neglected?

The process by which adaptation occurs also appears to need further research. The reward mechanism for "adaptors" is less defined than it is for "maintainers." The "maintainer" can rest assured that if, for example, the inventory level is adequate and the production line is operating smoothly, his job has been accomplished. The adaptor, however, must have a longer time horizon and the ability to live with considerable ambiguity. It seems clear, however, that the adaptor's role is critical—particularly in an organization whose environment is changing.

In general, the area of organizational adaptation in the public sector has received little attention. If we narrow the scope further to hospitals, we find even less research of quality has been done. According to Georgopoulos,[23] who attempted to summarize work in this area, research has tended to be below average quality. The best of what has been done is a study by Perrow,[24] who in 1971 looked at a 300-bed nonuniversity teaching hospital to inquire into the social conditions that affect organizational goals. The author saw hospitals' goals as the product of interaction between the hospital's social structure, leadership groups, and the environment as it is internally perceived.

In the same year, Elling and Halebsky[25] explored sponsorship and the receipt of support to study how an organization depends on its environment. In 1962, Rohrer[26] looked at trends in rural hospitals and found that they tend to change and are changed as their environment changes. A small number of additional studies are cited by Georgopoulos, but it would seem that some of the critical findings in the area of organizational behavior—particularly the work of Lawrence and Lorsch in industrial organizations—should be tested for their applicability to medical care organizations.

The Lawrence and Lorsch model[27] provides the most useful answer to the question of how adaptation occurs. A fundamental component of their model is that there is no one best way to organize, but that effective organizations develop structures that are congruent with the environments in which they operate. The authors postulate that complex environments necessitate variety in the number and kinds of units within the organization, each of which has specific tasks to perform in order to adequately respond to the environment. The extent of this division into manageable units, which Lawrence and Lorsch call "differentiation," is a function of certainty or uncertainty in the environment, the nature of the competition, and the diversity of the environment. They define the differentiation in terms of the formality of structure, interpersonal orientation, time, and goal orientation.

While it is useful for an organization to be composed of separate units in order to function effectively, it is also useful for some level of coordination to exist so that natural conflict resulting from different goals can be resolved. The authors propose that the higher the level of differentiation within an organization the more difficult it will be to effectively integrate the various units.

The problem becomes particularly complex in reference to multihospital health systems. Each hospital or unit within the system is made up of component parts that must operate separately and that tend to have different goals and different orientations. Yet they must collaborate when it comes to dealing with the product—improving health of a given patient. In a hospital system, this problem is especially true; the units that make up the system tend to have different goals and needs, and there also exists a need to work together at a system level. If one assumes, for purposes of discussion, that each hospital consists of three units—internal medicine, emergency room, and laboratory—each with its different time orientation and goals, then the problem can be represented as follows (Figure 4.1):

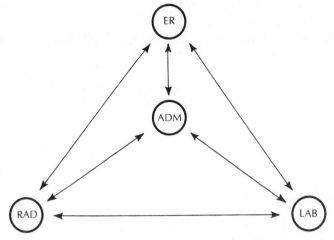

Figure 4.1. Component parts of a freestanding hospital.

When one adds the complexity of a system to the above, one has:

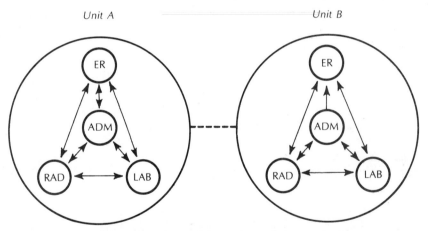

Figure 4.2. Component parts of a system.

This does not even present the added complexity of the arrows which often need to exist between, for example, the emergency room at Unit A with the labs at Unit B.

One of the essential components of the Lawrence and Lorsch model is an expanded view of organizational structure. Whereas the classicists envisioned the structure as "boxes on a chart," the contingency theorists see structures as a more inclusive phenomenon. While teams and committees do play a critical part in achieving the appropriate levels of differentiation and integration, it would seem to be the job of the leader and managers within the organization to assess what the "appropriate" level means.

The role of the leader in an autonomous institution is likely to be quite different than in a multihospital system because of the complexity previously discussed. The task of determining a stragety for the system—how it is to relate to its environment and how it should be designed in order to respond both to external demands and to the needs of its workers—largely falls to the chief executive officer and his staff. What, then, do we know about leadership within a complex system? These systems are aptly described by Forrester:[28]

> Complex systems have many important characteristics that we must understand if we expect to design systems with better behavior. Complex systems are counter-intuitive, are remarkably insensitive to changes in many systems parameters, stubbornly resist policy changes, contain influential pressure points (often in unexpected places) from which forces will radiate to alter system balance, counteract and compensate for externally applied corrective efforts by reducing the corresponding internally-generated action (the corrective program is largely absorbed in replacing lost internal action), often react to a policy change in the long run in a way opposite to how they react in the short run, tend toward low performance.

One might thus assume that complex systems by their very nature elude exploration. One can argue, however, that systematic exploration is possible and that it becomes critical to develop conceptual maps which can adequately describe the system in question.

The literature on how a complex system adapts, how it can be designed, and how it can be led, represent pieces of the "conceptual map" which lead to increased understanding of the multihospital system.

ORGANIZATIONAL LEADERSHIP

The concept of leadership remains elusive. If the consequences of different leadership processes could be regularly predicted within a given set of environmental constraints, then those tasks and processes could be chosen that best lead to preferred criteria. Unfortunately, available literature has not been predictive.

The literature on leadership is, however, extensive, if characterized by incohesiveness. There is no theory which purports to explain leadership behavior and, within the hospital setting, there has been little effort to identify what variables are linked to the effective development of the organization. Although much of the research on leadership has had as its theoretical base the study of the modern integrated firm rather than the more fragmented hierarchical structure of the hospital, there is a significant amount of research that can be applied to the leadership of the multihospital system.

Since research on leadership has lacked cohesion, it has consequently been difficult to apply because it has concentrated on individual variables that together rather than individually account for considerable differences in leadership.

We have, for example, considerable data on the *situation,* and on the *individual,* and little data about the interaction of the situation *with* the individual, or about how these interactions change as the organization matures.

We take for granted that an organization will thrive under competent leadership, and that it will fail or do considerably less well under poor leadership. Yet we know little about the factors that make leaders effective or ineffective. For the most part, judgments about the effectiveness of a leader are made not on the basis or *what* he does, but on the *visible effects* of what he does, such as the financial performance of the particular company. Yet it seems critical to understand the process by which decisions are made, the organizational structure, and especially the strategy the leader chooses to best achieve the organization's objectives.

In a nonprofit organization, it becomes especially important to understand what it is that the leader does or does not do, inasmuch as exterior measures of performance are considerably more difficult to ascertain. While the private concern usually has a hierarchy of authority and fairly clear boundaries between the organization, its competitors, and other power bases within the community, the hospital tends to have a less clear hierarchy, and rather murky boundaries. It is never completely clear at any given time where the hospital stands in its relationships. Its constituencies are varied, and may change from one day to the next; it may be in competition with another hospital one day and working with that same hospital the next. This is not to say that these differences are clear-cut. Unfortunately, while for-profit and not-for-profit organizations cannot be conveniently put in different categories, it is fair to say that many of the characteristics of a for-profit organization make it easier to explore the components of leadership.

The best evidence for my contention that leadership is more difficult to explore and evaluate in a nonprofit situation is that the concept is usually ignored in organizational research pertaining to hospitals. It is simply assumed that if the hospital is doing well it is being run effectively, and that when it stops being run effectively it will no longer do well. Outside the hospital area, however, concern with leadership has received a great deal of attention. During the past few decades, as tasks have become more complex and as the organization has been forced to deal with more outside institutions and to realize that it is part of an interdependent system, leadership has received considerably more attention, as it has become clear that somebody must take responsibility for coordinating the efforts of the complex organization.

Yet while it is understood that leadership is a significant aspect of human activity, research in the field has produced very little of use to the manager, either in the for-profit or nonprofit sector. To be sure, leadership research is plagued by a number of extremely difficult problems. Comparability of data is difficult to achieve. Leaders (even when they can easily be pinpointed) find it difficult to articulate their activities in a way that potential leaders may emulate or apply to their own organizations. When these activities are reduced to statistically significant units, such as number of superior/subordinate interactions or periods of time spent in meetings,[29] it becomes even more difficult to make the data useful to the person who is trying to become a good leader. Also, despite the intrinsic interest of the literature on leadership, it does not give institutions a great deal to work with when they want to choose the "right" leader from among available candidates.

Furthermore, all too often the terms leadership and managership are used interchangeably, and schools of management do not often seem clear as to what they can teach or are teaching. While definitions of a leader vary immensely (from the person who creates the most effective change in group performance to that person identified and accepted as leader by his followers), it seems reasonable for our purposes to make some preliminary definitions of leadership, to differentiate it from managing, and to begin to outline how leadership as a concept is useful in understanding the multihospital system.

I would suggest that managing refers to the efficient and effective solution of today's problems, while leadership is a far broader concept. The leader not only identifies the problems of immediate concern to the organization, but also identifies the areas that are not yet problems but that must be addressed today if they are to be effectively dealt with and not become problems. To do both of these, the leader must orchestrate people, facilities, and funds so that there is a clear strategy that is understood at the top level of the organization, whose parts are understood at other levels. The structure of the organization must reflect this strategy, and both the strategy and the structure must be flexible and reactive so that the organization can react to environmental demands before these demands become insurmountable obstacles.

These functions are particularly difficult in a health institution, where the boundaries are often not clear and where it is often even less clear who the members of the reporting structure are or how extensive is the leader's authority within the organization. The problems between medical staffs and administrators are legion, but if one adds to this the natural antagonisms between planners, regulators, trustees, and consumers (all of whom play a critical role in the leader's work, yet do not have a clear position on the organization chart), it becomes easier to see why the leader of a health organization plays such a complex role.

Studies of leadership often fall into the area of leadership style, which can be described as the visible aspect of the leadership process. Within this category, there are at least three groupings:

leadership style as a function of the leader's personality—the "Great Man" or "trait" school;
leadership style as a function of the interaction between the leader and subordinates—the "personal behavior" theory;
leadership style as a function of the situation's demands—the "contingency" theory.

The "Great Man" school describes leadership as a function of the leader's inborn or acquired traits. According to this theory, the manager's internal constraints determine how he will diagnose a situation and select the appropriate management behavior. And it is indeed true that many a leader puts his personal stamp on his organization. The leader of a psychiatric hospital in England, for example, gained an international reputation for giving the psychiatric nurses in his hospital's outpatient department nontraditional management roles. But psychiatrists on the hospital staff resented the leader's emphasis on nurses; their resignations led to the hospital's decline.

According to the Great Man school, the personality of the leader is the influence that shapes others' behavior so that it is consonant with the organization's goals. Trait theorists suggest that the best leader is someone who is superior in verbal facility, judgment, scholarship, I.Q., initiative, self-confidence, self-awareness, perceptiveness, ability to communicate, and even physical qualities such as stature. They tell us that the great man will choose from his personal repertory of behaviors the one most appropriate for specific situations. The implication is that there is one kind of personality, or constellation of personal traits, that is the best in all management situations.[30]

In contrast to the foregoing, the personal behaviorists define leadership as a function of the interaction between leaders and subordinates. While most leadership theories have viewed the leader in a rather detached manner, it seems clear that he acts and reacts in relation to other people with whom he comes in contact. Just as the leader has his own norms and expectations, background and values, so do other people in his group, whether or not they are in any way articulated. In point of fact, they are seldom articulated and even more seldom taken into account by the leader. Homans, of the interactionist school, developed a model of the human group that is useful in exploring the relationship of the leader to his subordinates.[31] According to this model, certain activities, interactions, and sentiments are essential for the group to accomplish its work. In other activities jobs must be performed that require people to work together, which Homans calls interactions. As people interact, they tend to develop certain attitudes or sentiments—either positive or negative—about one another. Positive sentiments can lead to new or emergent activities among group members, such as having lunch together. Negative sentiments can also emerge in the process of accomplishing the task, and these tend to lead to a disruptive climate, where no mutually supportive norms develop. An organization that is characterized by negative sentiments is likely to be unhealthy. If a leader were to take over such an organization, it is unlikely that he would realize the source of the dissatisfaction or understand the dynamics of the negative sentiments. Instead, he would be more likely to see the end results of such dysfunction—high absenteeism, unusual turnover, or low production.

Classical theorists paid little attention to issues such as these. In their view, the organization consisted of rational people who were primarily motivated by money and could be effectively managed by the use of a clear and unbroken chain of command. Weber, for example, discussed three types of authority in an attempt to characterize organizations in terms of the authority relationships within them.[32] He outlined three pure types which he labeled "charismatic," "traditional," and "rational legal." The latter describes the bureaucratic organizational form that Weber saw as the dominant institution of modern society. The system is reactional because the means are expressly designed to achieve certain specific goals. The organization is viewed as a well-designed machine with certain functions to perform, every part of whose machinery contributes to the attainment of maximum performance of that function. It is legal because authority is exercised by means of a system of rules and procedures through the office an individual occupies at a particular time.

Weber calls this organizational form a bureaucracy, which to him had a very different connotation than the modern connotation (which usually implies inefficiency and excessive attention to unimportant detail). To Weber, the bureaucracy was technically the most efficient form of organization possible. While the bureaucracy was like a modern machine, other organizational forms were like nonmechanical methods of production. The bureaucracy was, according to Weber, unencumbered by the personal whims of the leader. It represented the ultimate form of depersonalization—officials were arranged in a hierarchy, each successive step embracing all those beneath it, working according to a set of rules and procedures, within which each possible contingency is theoretically provided for.

Weber was by no means alone in his assumptions about the rationality of the bureaucracy, managed by experts and run with utmost efficiency. Chester Barnard, as chief executive at Bell Telephone, where the values of "service" and "duty" prevailed, believed that complex organizations exhibited regularities of structure and processes which could be reduced to "principles of administration." To Barnard, there was little problem regarding the role of the individual within the organization—by the very fact that he had been hired, the individual had granted authority to his superiors; when he was not willing to obey a superior, he would leave the organization.

The classical theorists, then, with few exceptions,[33] gave little attention to the problems of an unhealthy organization where individuals were not working to their fullest capacity. It was assumed that a well-run organization was possible. Consequently, problems that occurred at the personal and interpersonal levels could be avoided by competent management.

Modern theorists such as Schein, Argyris, Fiedler, and Vroom, on the other hand, have addressed the problem of working within a complex organization from the individual's point of view. To them, it is by no means obvious that personal and interpersonal problems can or should be avoided. They believe that the overall objective of the organization is to achieve a satisfactory integration between the needs and desires of its members and the persons functionally related to it, such as consumers, shareholders, and suppliers. Schein describes leadership within the framework of the contingency theory.[34] His "complex man" first diagnoses the needs of people, groups, tasks, organizational structures, and environment, and then chooses leadership behavior that will move the organization towards its predetermined goals. The situation dictates the behavior—subject, of course, to some modification by the leader's own predilections. Argyris, Vroom, and Fiedler[35] are all concerned with how the quality of leadership can be improved in organizational settings. However, their definitions of leadership vary considerably, as do their prescriptions for overall improvement in organizational leadership.

Argyris emphasizes the "reeducation" of managers to move from one set of behavior strategies to another. He considers this process to be of significant benefit for both the leader and the organization. Argyris calls these behaviors Models 1 and 2, and focuses on developing skills that enable the leader to increase his effectiveness. His assumption is that organizations are dysfunctional in that they are counterproductive to individual growth and that, in order for the individual to influence effectively (which is Argyris's definition of leadership), he must learn the difference between what he believes and what he actually does. Thus, Argyris devises experimental settings in which subjects become deeply involved over long periods of time and are eventually able to transfer the knowledge to the noncontrived world. He admits that changing behavior is a time-consuming and painful process, but he is optimistic about the ability of managers to learn and thus to influence more effectively.

Fiedler, on the other hand, focuses on the effective diagnosis of the situation in which the leader will operate. He stresses the matching of the leader to the situation, which involves either assigning the leader to the situation that is appropriate to his basic personality or changing the situation to fit the leader. Fiedler is less interested than Argyris in changing the leader; he concentrates instead on analyzing and changing the situation, being rather pessimistic about the possibility of training leaders. Fiedler begins by measuring the leader's motivation and goes on to divide his subjects into task-oriented and interpersonally oriented leaders. He has found in repeated studies that high relationship motivated leaders will generally perform best in situations which are moderately favorable, while task-oriented leaders tend to perform best in situations which are highly favorable or highly unfavorable. Fiedler believes that, while it is theoretically possible to change a person's motivational structure—the basic goals he pursues—it is considerably easier to change the leadership situation.

Vroom focuses on the development of a prescriptive decisionmaking model for leaders, one that is limited to the extent to which the leader should encourage subordinates to participate in the decisionmaking process. His work is somewhat more specific than that of Fiedler or Argyris, and he concentrates on helping leaders understand their natural tendencies. His model includes various situational variables, such as the amount of information available, relevant time constraints, and the necessity of acceptance.

Selznick's contribution to the research on leadership is also useful. He begins by asking how organizational change is produced, and how it shapes the interaction of individuals. He then argues that true leadership occurs when the transition is made from administrative management to institutional leadership, thus differentiating an organization from an institution. The former is designed as a:

. . . technical instrument for mobilizing human energies and directing them toward set aims. We allocate tasks, delegate authority, channel communication, and find some say of coordinating all that has been divided up and parcelled out. All this is conceived as an exercise in engineering; it is governed by the related ideals of rationality and discipline.[36]

An institution, on the other hand, "is more nearly a product of social needs and pressures—a responsive, adaptive organism."[37] The process by which an organization becomes an institution is a gradual one: "It is something that happens to an organization over time, reflecting the organization's own distinctive history, the people who have been in it, the groups it embodies and the vested interests they have created, and the way it has adapted to its environment."[38]

This process of change is within the purview of the leader, whose job it is to "infuse [the organization] with value" beyond the technical requirements of the task at hand. Thus, for Selznick, the nature of leadership does not vary with each social situation; significant leadership patterns are relatively few.

It would seem that the CEO of a modern organization cannot ignore the problems that are bound to occur within a complex organization. Before he can address these problems, however, he must know what assumptions he makes about the people who work for him. Just as all organizational theorists make certain assumptions about individuals, so every leader has similar assumptions that affect every aspect of his job, and which form the basis of his leadership style and lead him to a decision about which tasks will be addressed and how the organization will relate to its larger environment.

While most reasearchers have concentrated on management style in an effort to differentiate among leaders, style is an amalgam of the assumptions that a leader makes, and it is these assumptions which have the most far-reaching organizational reverberations. It is understandable that style has received so much attention, since it is far more accessible than the assumptions upon which the style is based. The research on management style has primarily consisted of descriptive dichotomies which view behavior in two ways: it either emphasizes attention to the task at hand, or to people whose job it is to accomplish the task. A review of the literature in this area yields a veritable plethora of "alphabetical" dichotomies, many of which shed light on the assumptions made by the leader.

McGregor,[39] for example, suggested that there are two different sets of assumptions about human nature and human motivation. One set of assumptions, which he called Theory X, suggests that people are basically lazy, unreliable, and irresponsible, motivated only by what Maslow calls the "lower level physiological and safety needs"; therefore, the only way one gets anything [out of them] in a work situation is to direct, control, and closely supervise their behavior. Theory Y's assumptions, on the other hand, reflect a more positive view of people. They could be creative and self-directed at work if properly motivated at the higher social, esteem, and self-actualization need levels, as described by Maslow.

Argyris in his earlier work[40] identified behavior patterns A and B, which generally correspond with Theories X and Y. Pattern A represents leader behavior characterized by close supervision, a high degree of structure, and "telling" behavior; Pattern B, according to Argyris, is characterized by general supervision, high consideration, and "participating" behavior. As Argyris emphasized, while XA and YB are usually associated with each other, they need not be under certain circumstances; Pattern A could go with Theory Y or Pattern B with Theory X. Blake[41] proposes a two-dimensional typology: "more" or "less" concern with tasks and "more" or "less" concern with people, each measured on a scale of one to nine. Tannenbaum and Schmidt[42] propose a boss–subordinate approach that measures the extent to which a manager is prepared to delegate authority. Both approaches suggest some important dimensions of behavior, but do not describe situations in which specific behaviors are appropriate.

The difficulty of having one set of assumptions about people is that all too often they become self-fulfilling prophecies. If individuals are treated as if they are lazy and unreliable, and are therefore always told what to do and when to do it, they will gradually begin to behave as if they were that kind of person. This can become a downward spiralling effect, whereby low expectations produce even lower productivity.

Besides dichotomies of approach such as the ones established by Argyris and McGregor, as well as by Likert and Blake and Mouton, there are also a number of descriptive terms which attempt to explain the way a leader behaves as an outward sign of the assumptions that he is making. Etzioni, for example, discusses the difference between position power and personal power. His distinction springs from the concept of power as the ability to induce or influence behavior. He claims that power is derived from an organizational office, personal influence, or both. Individuals who are able to induce another individual to do a certain job because of their position in the organization are considered to have position power; individuals who derive their power from their followers are considered to have personal power.

It is, of course, possible for some individuals to have both personal and position power. While position power is in a sense directly related to the job within the organization, personal power is much more far-reaching. It is unlikely for the janitor to have significant position power, but certainly plausible that he may have considerable personal power because of his ability to cultivate relationships with a number of people who do have position power and thus are in a position to extend his base. Examples of secretaries that "run the office" and telephone operators that can "make anything happen" are legion.

If a leader makes no effort to develop personal power and instead relies solely on his position power, he is usually making certain assumptions about people—that do not need to be motivated except by the most basic safety and physical needs, that increasing his interactions with them will not lead to a smoother working relationship with them, or that regardless of his actions his subordinates are not really willing or capable of change.

A number of researchers have explored leadership behavior as opposed to leadership traits and inherent skills. Foremost among these researchers is Mintzberg[43] who dissected the top manager's job into various components. He studied five executives in depth and described the content of their work, making an attempt to describe the "purpose" of each of the events observed. He later established what he called "content categories." He used concept of role and found that the manager had ten separate roles, ranging from figurehead to entrepreneur.

There have been a number of studies of this type that attempt to analyze the job of the manager. Neustadt analyzed Presidential power with particular reference to the immense set of forces acting on the officeholder. He studied three men who held the office in an effort to understand how these men had attained the personal power that characterized the office of the President.[44]

There also have been a number of significant empirical studies of managerial work based on the work diary. Perhaps the most comprehensive is that of Sune Carlson, who analyzed the work of nine Swedish directors who were asked to record their daily activities in diaries. His principal finding was that these executives viewed "getting information" as their single most difficult recurring task. Rosemary Taylor carried out another major diary study, in which she studied 160 senior and middle managers for four weeks each with the aim of discovering similarities and differences in the way managers spend their time. She attempted to achieve comparability of data, and reported her findings in the form of amounts of time spent at various tasks. She concluded that there were five job profiles that characterize all the executives she studied.

One of the most interesting pieces of research on managerial behavior was done by Hodgson, Levinson and Zaleznick, who studied the three senior executives of a large psychiatric hospital. Their research was based on intensive observation of the executives and their environment, with particular emphasis on personality and interpersonal behavior rather than on the work they did per se. The authors found that the roles that needed to be played within the organization were shared by the three executives in a "role constellation."[45] The work is particularly interesting in that it suggests that a variety of administrative forms are likely to be found in different organizations, ranging from the patriarchal to the diadic and triadic forms of leadership.

SUMMARY

Each of these areas of the literature adds information about the pattern of development which characterizes an MHS. Each area reviewed includes a large number of factors, only some of which are directly applicable to system development.

The literature on the MHS, for example, covers a broad range of variables, most of which are very specific, including legal bonds and the nature of combined services. Several factors emerge that appear useful in characterizing the seven systems studied: the history or tradition of collaboration in the area, the influence of pressure groups that can affect the kinds of activities that a system decides to emphasize, and the location of member units. In terms of the activities themselves, which comprise the system's response to external demands, the literature is considerably less useful.

The literature on the growth and development of organizations introduces the idea of specific stages characterized by specific activities and implies that managerial behavior is of particular importance when it is coupled with environmental assessment and corporate reactions to the results of such assessment.

The literature on organizational adaptation addresses the natural tendency of an organization to remain closed and also addresses the idea that, as the number of environmental factors that impinge on an organization grows, new organizational responses are necessary. In other words, in an increasingly complex world, organizations must become more complex.

In order to achieve an appropriate level of complexity, adaptive organizations often develop subsystems or units that are designed to perform specific functions in order to allow the organization to achieve its overall objectives.

The literature on leadership is diverse and includes such factors as an analysis of time spent by leaders performing certain activities, inborn traits such as verbal facility, judgment, and leadership style defined as an interaction between the leader and his subordinates. This body of leadership literature becomes more useful when the leader is viewed in relation to his organization. Weber, for example, postulated that in a bureaucracy, well structured rules and procedures negate the need for a leader. The modern theorists, particularly Schein, Argyris, Fiedler, and Vroom, deal with the leader as someone who can be trained to more effectively diagnose internal and external needs so that an organization can move towards predetermined goals. This interaction between the leader, his organization, and external demands, seems particularly useful.

Reviewing these areas provides a large number of factors that can be used to analyze the development of MHSs. What is particularly relevant is that interaction of the various areas, the relationship of the CEO or leader to the abilities of the organization to change in response to changes in external demands, and the nature of these demands. The linkages among these component parts are useful in better understanding the development of MHSs.

NOTES

1. James P. Cooney et al., *Multihospital Systems: An Evaluation, Part 2: Organizational Studies* (Health Services Research Center of the Hospital Research and Educational Trust and Northwestern University, 1975).
2. D. Rutstein, *The Coming Revolution in Medicine* (Cambridge, Mass.: M.I.T. Press, 1967).
3. M. Brown and H. Lewis, *Hospital Management Systems: Multi-Unit Organization and Delivery of Health Care* (Germantown, Md.: Aspen Systems Corporation, 1976).
4. AHA, p. 2.
5. Brown and Lewis, *Hospital Management Systems*, p. 30. There is a discrepancy between Brown's figure of 32 percent and a figure of 75 percent that was previously quoted. The difference is due to a definition of a "system."
6. E. Rostow, *Stages of Economic Growth.*
7. Alfred D. Chandler, *Strategy and Structure* (Cambridge, Mass.: M.I.T. Press, 1961).
8. Bruce R. Scott, *Stages of Corporate Development: A Descriptive Model* (Boston: Harvard Business School, ICCH #13G372, 1972).
9. Alfred Chandler, *The Visible Hand: The Managerial Revolution in American Business* (Cambridge, Mass.: Belknap Press, 1977).
10. Larry Greiner, "Evolution and Revolution as Organizations Grow," *Harvard Business Review,* July–August 1972.
11. Particularly by James March and Herbert Simon, *Organizations* (New York: Wiley, 1958); Tom Burns and G. M. Stalker, *The Management of Innovation* (London: Tavistock Publications and Social Science Paperback, 1966); James D. Thompson, *Organizations in Action* (New York: McGraw-Hill, 1967).

12. W. Ross Ashby, *Design for a Brain* (London: Chapman & Hall, Ltd., and Science Paperbacks, 1965).
13. This relates well to Schein's (1972) idea that the organization must be of use to its prime beneficiary.
14. N. A. Harvey, "Cybernetic Applications in Medicine. I. Medical Model Making," *New York Journal of Medicine*, March 15, 1965.
15. Chester I. Barnard, *The Functions of the Executive* (Cambridge, Mass.: Harvard University Press, 1938), p. 73.
16. Daniel Katz and R. L. Kahn, *The Social Psychology of Organization* (New York: Wiley, 1966), p. 31.
17. Nicos P. Mouzelis, *Organization and Bureaucracy: An Analysis of Modern Theories* (Chicago: Aldine, 1968).
18. R. Bales, "In Conference," *Harvard Business Review*, March–April, 1954.
19. Thompson, *Organizations in Action.*
20. Richard Harris, *A Sacred Trust* (New York: New American Library, 1966), p. 2.
21. March and Simon, *Organizations;* Richard Cyert and James March, *A Behavioral Theory of the Firm* (Englewood Cliffs, N.J.: Prentice-Hall, 1963).
22. Leslie A. Hart, *How the Brain Works* (New York: Basic Books, 1975).
23. Basil Georgopoulos, *Hospital Organization Research: Review and Source* (Philadelphia: Saunders Series in Health Care Organization and Administration, 1975).
24. Charles Perrow, *Organizational Analysis: A Sociological View* (London: Tavistock Publications, 1970).
25. R. H. Elling and S. Halebsky, "Organizational Differentiation and Support," *Administrative Science Quarterly* 6:2, 1971, p. 185.
26. W. C. Rohrer, "Demographic and Social Changes Affecting the Community Hospital," *Hospital Administration*, 1962, p. 32.
27. Paul R. Lawrence and Jay W. Lorsch, *Studies in Organizational Design* (Homewood, Ill.: Irwin & Dorsey, 1970).
28. Jay Forrester, *World Dynamics* (Cambridge, Mass.: Wright–Allen Press, 1971).
29. Henry Mintzberg, "The Manager—Folklore and Myth," *Harvard Business Review* (July–August, 1975).
30. Alan Sheldon and Diana Barrett, "The Janus Principle," *Health Care Management Review*, Spring 1977.
31. George Homans, *The Human Group* (New York: Harcourt Brace, 1950).
32. Max Weber, *The Theory of Social and Economic Organization* (New York: The Free Press, 1947).
33. Follett was unique in that she "wanted a better oriented society in which the individual could live a fuller and more satisfactory life," and she endeavored to find the "real avenue to this fuller life." M. P. Follett, in *Dynamic Administration*, H. C. Metcalf and L. Urwick (eds.), (New York: Harper & Row, 1942).
34. Edgar H. Scheip, *Organizational Psychology* (Englewood Cliffs, N.J.: Prentice-Hall, 1970).
35. Fiedler, Vroom and Argyris, *Organizational Dynamics, Leadership Symposium*, published by American Management Association.
36. Selznick, *Leadership in Administration*, p. 5.
37. Ibid., p. 16.
38. Ibid.
39. D. McGregor, *The Human Side of Enterprise* (New York: McGraw-Hill, 1960).
40. Chris Argyris and D. Schon, *Theory in Practice: Increasing Professional Effectiveness* (San Francisco: Jossey-Bass, 1974).

41. R. R. Blake, *The Grid for Sales Excellence* (with J. S. Mouton) (New York: McGraw-Hill, 1970).
42. R. Tannenbaum and W. Schmidt, "How to Choose a Leadership Pattern," *Harvard Business Review,* May–June 1973.
43. Henry Mintzberg, *The Nature of Managerial Work* (New York: Harper & Row, 1973).
44. R. Neustadt, "Presidential Power," in *The Politics of Leadership* (New York: Wiley, 1960).
45. R. C. Hodgson, D. J. Levinson, and A. Zaleznick, *The Executive Role Constellation* (Boston: Division of Research, Harvard Business School, 1965).

Chapter 5

Profiles of Sites and Chief Executive Officers

INTRODUCTION

As we have seen, a variety of collaborative forms exist among health institutions. We have explored the regulatory and financial pressures which encourage collaboration and we have addressed the various forms of collaboration. Whether the collaboration takes place spontaneously or reactively in an effort to avoid further pressure, and regardless of the form of collaboration in question, there are certain issues that are common to all multihospital systems and that must be addressed as the system matures.

It is difficult to define each of the seven systems studied as a "type." If one thinks in terms of a spectrum of cooperation ranging from the most informal alliance around a given issue—such as cooperative purchasing—to a complex relationship in which each institution can both provide service and purchase service, each system would have a unique place in the spectrum. Each of the systems studied came about as a result of extremely different environmental peculiarities, and is structured and organized very differently. One might, for example, characterize both the St. John's Hospital and Homes system and the

Note: All names and places have been fictionalized.

Springvale Hospital System as satellite systems. Yet this description gives little sense to the other factors which differentiate them, such as the issue of geographical proximity, one's having come about as a result of a legislative act while the other was founded by religious laymen to serve rural areas that could not efficiently manage their own hospitals. It is for this reason that I have not put labels on the different sites, and instead have attempted to describe them in depth so that the development of each system can be better understood.

Brief profiles of each site and of each chief executive officer will be presented to give the reader an overall picture of the seven sites. The data will then be discussed in the next chapter.

MID–ATLANTIC REGIONAL HOSPITALS

The Mid-Atlantic Regional Hospitals (MARH) was established in 1963 as a nonprofit corporation to run five hospitals in eastern states. These hospitals had originally been established to serve the needs of miners and had been run by the Miners Memorial Hospital Association. It became increasingly difficult to manage these institutions as the cost of care rose and as these financial problems threatened the fiscal integrity of the United Mine Workers' fund. An appeal by the president of the United Mine Workers (UMW) of America to the Board of Missions of the United Church of Christ resulted in the formation of MARH.

The MARH today includes ten hospitals, each with an emergency room and an outpatient clinic. Eight of the facilities provide home health care and there are extended care facilities at four hospitals. The system attempts to be responsive to the health needs as well as the illness needs of the population and to be comprehensive in scope. As a result, it has been in financial distress since its inception. The managerial strategy has generally been to involve the communities heavily in the operation of the hospitals and to decentralize a system that has been highly centralized. Financial problems worsened considerably during 1977, as the combination of an extreme winter, followed by floods and the threat of strike, led to a loss of 8,000 patient-days. As a result, the system is dangerously close to having to drastically curtail its services. In addition, the UMW decreased its benefits, and rather than sending the system the unexpected $1.4 million in July of that year, sent it less than half that amount, worsening an already critical situation. Dr. Dyer, a surgeon and researcher who became the system's president in 1972, has appealed to HEW for moneys in the form of a demonstration grant in order to keep the system intact.

The system is unique in that it is based on outreach efforts that tend to be financial liabilities. There are about 150 four-wheeled vehicles that travel the mountains carrying home health aids, pediatric nurse practitioners, physicians' assistants, and health education specialists. Distances are significant between facilities, and of course affect the costs of the services delivered. The MARH has permanent facilities in eighteen communities, including the ten hospitals, the corporate office, a central management services group, and two outreach stations. The system is governed by means of a thirty-three-member central board as well as by local governing boards.

The CEO

Dr. Donald Dyer is the CEO at Mid-Atlantic Regional Hospitals. A surgeon and a research scientist, he took over the leadership of an organization that had been closely managed by Joseph C. Martin, who retired in 1975. The organization was then, and still is, in serious financial trouble, and Dr. Dyer's tenure has been marked by a constant need to reassess the mission of the system in light of economic realities.

Dr. Dyer was active in the Church of Christ Missions and originally became involved with MARH to see whether it was feasible for the Church to take over the system. It did not make sense for it to do so, but Dyer was put on the MARH board in 1963 and became chairman ten years later. He has strong opinions about what the system should try to be—a "health" rather than an "illness" system—for he feels most MHSs deal with crisis intervention and illness care. His system, however, is oriented toward keeping people healthy. But it is difficult to implement this philosophy, which is expensive, when the UMW reduces miners' benefits as drastically as it recently did, and consequently reduces the funds it gives the hospital system. In July of 1977, rather than receiving the expected annual payment of $1.4 million to run the system, MARH received $470,000, making it necessary to either close significant parts of the system, or find a new source of funds.

Dr. Dyer likes to think in terms of goals and targets, which he often sets for himself. When he came to MARH, he set four objectives that he wanted to meet: (1) to find the causes of the system's problems; (2) to reorganize the system so that it would run more efficiently, and at the same time serve the large, indigent population; (3) to make it cost effective; and (4) to make it financially sound. He feels that the first three have been accomplished, but given the extremely severe winter of 1976, floods, a strike, and the recent decrease in funds, it does not seem likely that the fourth objective will be met.

He likes to work with a small staff. When he arrived, there were five vice presidents; one left, and he eventually fired two others. He depends on what he considers to be a sophisticated management information system. Dr. Dyer seems fairly comfortable working with this system at a time of crisis and wants to see it through.

HILLCREST COMMUNITY HOSPITALS

Hillcrest Community Hospitals, in the Midwest, is a nonprofit, multiple-unit hospital system that both owns its own hospitals and manages them. Its chief executive officer, Wayne Garrett, both writes and speaks often about the holding company concept, which is at the base of the Hillcrest system.

Garrett defines the bank holding company as any company that has ownership control over a bank or group of banks with a central corporate office. He believes, however, that the individual member banks must maintain their own boards in order to respond to community needs, and he carries this analogy of the holding company to the hospital field.

The Hillcrest system traces its history to 1905 when a group of Finnish pastors and laymen founded the Finnish United Church Hospital Corporation. Within a few years they had acquired a large site on the banks of the Mississippi River, and began construction that year on a tuberculosis facility. By 1914, the corporation had changed its name to United Church Hospital Association and had enough money to add two wings to the existing institution. Several years later, Hillcrest Lutheran Hospital opened, and it has been growing ever since. In the early 1970s the word Lutheran was dropped from the hospital name.

Today, the 415-bed Hillcrest Hospital is located in a highly institutionalized community, which includes the 493-bed St. Ann's Hospital as well. The hospital jointly operates two family practice clinics in conjunction with St. Ann's and the university medical school. Hillcrest also operates an extensive rehabilitation center, a 75-bed extended care facility, and is constructing a medical office building in conjunction with St. Ann's. In 1965, Hillcrest–Willowdale Hospital was opened in a growing suburban area; it was expanded three years later to keep up with the population demands. The opening of Hillcrest–Willowdale marked the beginning of a multiple unit system. Eight years later, in 1973, a third unit, Memorial Hospital, joined the system. This particular hospital is located in the inner city where many residents are American Indians; thus outpatient care is emphasized, and a number of services are directed specifically at this population. At the present time, the system owns and operates the 405-bed Hillcrest Hospital, the 402-bed Hillcrest–Willowdale Hospital, the 250-bed Memorial Hospital, the 35-bed Harbridge Community Hospital, and the Downtown Health Center. Altogether, there are a total of 1,092 acute beds. In addition, the system manages the Nichols Area Memorial Hospital, and has an affiliation agreement with ten other area hospitals. The Hillcrest management is available as a consulting team to the area institutions who can use their expertise without submerging their own identities. The system has both capability and experience in dealing with varied community groups, and is using this background to develop a 140-acre site over the next fifteen years that will include a new Lutheran church, an outpatient clinic, a facility for the aging population in the area, and a doctors' office building.

The Hillcrest system is governed by a twenty-five-member board of trustees. Garrett and administrators of the corporate-owned hospitals are board members. Hillcrest, Hillcrest–Willowdale, and Memorial have, however, retained their own boards, as well as separate medical staffs.

The CEO

Wayne Garrett, the CEO at Hillcrest Community Hospitals, originally wanted to be a physician. But, he says, "I loved the medical environment, but I was terrible in the sciences. So with my degree in social psychology, it seemed a natural fit. I studied hospital administration in graduate school, and I've been happy ever since."

While in graduate school, Garrett was an administrative assistant and an administrative resident at Chicago's Northwestern Hospital. He was assistant administrator there after graduation. When he accepted the position as administrator of Hillcrest Hospital in 1952, the position had been open for nearly a year. "Nobody else wanted it," he says. In 1963, Garrett became executive vice president of Hillcrest. In 1970, he was named president of the Hillcrest Hospitals, and in 1973, president of Hillcrest Community Hospitals.

Garrett's career has developed within the Hillcrest system. He is by nature a builder and a developer rather than a manager, although he has surrounded himself with a first-rate management team that insulates him from the day-to-day operational problems of the system and frees him to deal with growth opportunities. His general attitude toward administration is to provide physicians with planning, an efficient environment, and quality control, and to use his own time to work as a regional and national proponent for the system's concept.

Since 1971 he has championed the idea of the hospital holding concept, which in effect means that individual units, like bank branches, have autonomy by means of local boards, which can remain responsive to local demands. According to him, "Boards are going to have to look beyond the psychology of the single roof. If they don't look at the total community health care needs, they will default and the proprietaries will move in."

Hillcrest, with Garrett at its helm, has advanced steadily from $1.6 million assets, a single facility, and 178 beds in 1952 to the present form of a $60 million multihospital system. Garrett is a gregarious man who looks as if he would be perfectly comfortable as a director of a major bank or at an investment banking house on Wall Street. He seems comfortable as a national figure, and speaks proudly of his receipt of honors from the Finnish government.

THE SPRINGVALE HOSPITAL SYSTEM

The Springvale Hospital System is a vertically and horizontally integrated organization of nine facilities and 1,107 beds located in a southern state. It is both an urban and a rural system that was established in 1947 by an act of the state's General Assembly. This act, passed during a time when Springvale County was experiencing a surge of population growth, provided for "the establishment of an independent, self-perpetuating board of trustees to govern and operate the hospital as a community, nonprofit, voluntary institution on behalf of all citizens of Springvale County." At that time there was one hospital, which officially became a system in 1952 when citizens of Endicott, a community about twelve miles northeast of the center city, petitioned for a hospital, which led to the construction of the twenty-seven-bed George Herman Memorial Hospital.

There are presently three divisions, each managed by an administrator. The general division has day-to-day responsibility for the 430-bed Springvale General Hospital located in the center of the city. This division also has management control over the Weiss Center for Family Medicine, the site of a family practice residency program. A suburban division has responsibility for four facilities: the 110-bed George Herman Memorial Hospital at Endicott, the 80-bed Donald Larsen Nursing Center, a long-term facility also at Endicott; the 50-bed Morton Hospital, and the 29-bed North Springvale Hospital. The newest operating unit is called the center division because it is located near the geographical center of the county. Most of the major development, including a new tertiary care center, is located here. The facilities are the 307-bed Springvale Memorial Hospital that will be expanded to

700 beds by 1980; the 50-bed Irene C. Randolph Institute of Rehabilitative Medicine, and the 50-bed Francis L. Lantz Hospital that concentrates on psychiatric care. All the units are located within a thirty minute drive of one another. The SHS institutions are supported by a Management Services Center where personnel, fiscal programs, and filing and data processing are centralized, and a supply and distribution center. There are also three non-SHS hospitals in the county: the 60-bed Community Hospital for Crippled Children; the 195-bed Saint Joseph Community Hospital, and the 79-bed Slater Memorial Hospital.

SHS is governed by seven trustees who are charged to make overall policy. Three members reside in the city, three live outside the city but in the county, and one is an at-large member. This reflects the establishment of the SHS, whereby the city ceded its property and hospital to an independent board set up by state law and created for that purpose. The county matched the value of the city property with cash. The commissioners serve six-year terms; new members are approved by the city and the county governing units. The general director, Craig Gardner, reports to the trustees and is responsible for external relations and development, the Treasurer's office, and community services. Jack Fisher reports to Gardner and is responsible for the three hospital divisions and institutional support services. There is an open medical staff whereby doctors work within clinical departments, but they can cross institutional lines to treat any patient in any SHS facility.

Expansion, which has kept up with population shifts and growth, has been funded as a result of a referendum for a constitutional amendment in 1966 that allowed the system to incur a debt not exceeding 25 percent of the assessed property valuation in the county. Over the years, the SHS has used funds from a variety of other sources to finance capital projects. About 40 percent of its money has come from sources outside the county; the other 60 percent has been supplied by a $22 million bond issue made in 1968 and 1969, and $30 million in bonds authorized for the current development program. In July 1976, the SHS offered $7 million in tax exempt bonds for sale as the initial financing phase of the new bond issue. This money will allow an expansion of Springvale Memorial to 700 beds. A mental health center also will be built at the Seaver Road site, a 147-acre campus that should prove adequate for future expansion.

It is interesting to note that while consolidation of existing facilities and the construction of new ones has occurred, this system is unique in that it began as a system, and has not had to address the political complexities of bringing together units that have been autonomous for a number of years. The SHS has forged and maintained strong links to its communities by means of four fifteen–member Community Advisory Councils, representing the county's four service areas, named in 1974. Councils meet monthly, and are urged to advise the leadership concerning the needs and problems of their own areas.

The SHS is located in a prosperous area with a diversified economic base. An important interstate highway, which connects three major metropolitan areas, runs through the Springvale area. There is a high level of industrial activity throughout the area.

In 1974, the eight facilities had 39,709 admissions and provided 292,683 adult days of care.

The CEO

Craig Gardner is unique among the chief executive officers studied in that he has always worked in a hospital system. His first job was administrator of three hospitals in New York State that were established through philanthropic contributions from the founder of a major drug chain. "He assumed that if it worked for drugstores, it ought to work for hospitals." From there, Gardner went to a major hospital in New York City. "I made some mistakes and created some problems in the attempt to bring these three communities together—learned that it's very difficult to meld two different county medical societies, to change referral patterns, and to create a system of medical care as well as institutional care." Gardner was asked to go to Springvale and operate a hospital which would soon double in size, and so in January, 1953, he arrived there just as it became clear that a satellite unit was needed. From that time he has overseen the growth of the Springvale Hospital System.

His graduate training was in hospital administration in New York and in education in Massachusetts. He hypothesizes that it was this combination that "makes me look upon myself as an institutional manager rather than a hospital administrator, and it really works. . . . It seemed to me, and it still does, that whether I was running a long-term, short-term, acute rehabilitative or nursing institution, my mission was to provide clinically and geographically decentralized facilities with a coordinated and centralized management service to operate them.

Gardner has had the opportunity to build a system from the beginning, which has given him the freedom to innovate and give himself the time to assess changing needs and respond to them.

He has become a national figure, serving as a member of an American Hospital Association committee, and he is viewed as a philosopher in the health care field. Gardner and his staff, who handle the day-to-day operations, have built a system that has strong citizen input and solid backing from local and state government.

ST. JOHN'S HOSPITALS AND HOMES SOCIETY

St. John's Hospitals and Homes Society (SJHHS) is the largest nongovernmental not-for-profit multiple hospital system in the United States. It operates ninety institutions in sixty-five communities in thirteen western and midwestern states. These facilities include fifty-seven hospitals, twenty-four skilled nursing homes, six intermediate care facilities, two homes for the aged, and a school for crippled children. Twenty-nine of the institutions are owned by the society and the remainder are operated through lease agreements with the ownership body.

The system was established in 1938 by a group of Episcopalian laymen, who chose Michael Howard as executive director so that he might apply his previous experience as business manager for mission outposts to the failing hospitals. The system today is unique in its ability to function in such diverse environments. It is governed by a sixteen-member board of Episcopalian laymen, which is independent of the administrative staff; in fact, Clarence Coleman, president and chief executive officer, is not a member of the board.

All the institutions are managed as if they were owned; there are no "categories" of membership. The centralized services of the society's home office are utilized by each institution using identical procedures, reducing the need for personnel in each unit.

The system is unique as a rural health system organized in such a way that small hospitals can survive and flourish. Each institution has its own community board of directors appointed by the society's board, and the medical staff of each institution is directly responsible to the society's board, but the local board processes applications, outlines privileges, and makes recommendations for action to the society's board of directors.

At present, a large building program is underway. In early 1976, the society had $60 million in new construction in progress involving nine major projects in six states. The capital to finance this growth is obtained in a number of ways, generally by tax-exempt revenue bonds which have sold easily. The system is strong financially, with a $14 million line of credit with a consortium of banks.

The CEO

Clarence Coleman is the CEO of a ninety-one-unit rural-based system with headquarters in Minnesota. In 1948, Coleman had just left the service and joined what had until that time been known as the Twelve Apostles System. The system was then run by Michael Howard, an Episcopalian missionary, and had a gross volume of 900,000. Coleman started as assistant to Howard. He knew little about hospitals, but "Howard offered to give me half of what I had been getting teaching history and music and offered to teach me how to run hospitals from the bottom up. I did bookkeeping, I did maintenance, I even learned how to fire the boiler." At the beginning the arrangement worked very informally, with first Howard and then Coleman traveling around the country doing the bookkeeping for all the rural hospitals. "We'd collect all the sheets, add up all the number of receipts they had, and pay all the bills without even having an adding machine."

This early training characterizes the way Coleman works today. He still believes in learning from "the bottom up," and is in a sense still running the same kind of shop, although the level of sophistication has increased dramatically. Earnings have gone from $900,000 to $100 million, making one of his main roles right now that of financier. The system is unique in that it is a rurally based system, which involves travel over great distances for Coleman, his two vice presidents, and the field administrators. The closest facility is eighty miles from the corporate headquarters; the farthest is in Fairbanks, Alaska, several thousand miles away. A critical task for Coleman has been that of maintaining community autonomy and responsibility for an institution while at the same time providing corporate direction and expertise.

Coleman is musically oriented and uses musical metaphors often in his speech. This, coupled with the exterior appearance of someone who could be a country storekeeper but is running an enormous system that is still growing at an impressive rate, provides an interesting anomaly.

WESTERN AFFILIATED HOSPITAL SOCIETY

The Western Affiliated Hospital Society is a large not-for-profit MHS with a for-profit subsidiary called California Health Management Services. As the society developed expertise in management techniques, Jesse Lorrimer, the chief executive officer, developed the spinoff to capitalize on this expertise.

Western Affiliated Hospital Society (WAHS) was founded in 1920 by a group of Methodist laymen. The health care program remained small until 1940, when a second hospital was acquired. Today, the hospital owns two hospitals, manages five others on a lease basis, and has strong shared services and management ties to an eighth hospital. After California Health Management Services was begun in 1975, the corporation's central service functions were shifted into this subsidiary, including data processing accounting, construction and design, management engineering, planning, and public relations. In addition to California Health Management Services (CHMS), there is also a nonprofit cooperative called Western Medical Management Cooperative, which deals with all the hospital operations and management relationships. There are separate boards of directors for the cooperative and for the management company as well as for the society itself. The latter remains at least 51 percent Methodist. There are two classes of membership in the cooperative—one category for those institutions that purchase full services from the management company, and one for those that purchase only certain specific services. The former—those institutions owned or managed by the cooperative—have the benefit of sharing any profits.

The objective of establishing these nonprofit subsidiaries was to maintain the benefits inherent in a community hospital and the philosophy of WAHS and still compete with other management and shared services corporations by turning a profit.

At the present time, the society is involving itself in consulting and attempting to develop more volume by expanding its client base. Recent clients have included industrial concerns as well as area hospitals who want to use the services of the society to save money through shared services and sophisticated management expertise. The society is also considering working in conjunction with other regional MHSs such as Sun State Health Service to provide shared services.

The CEO

Jesse Lorrimer, the CEO of the Western Affiliated Hospital Society, has been a proponent of the MHS for many years. "I have preached this sort of thing for years, saying 'This is the only way to go.' But people don't want to change until they have to. And I think they find out now that you're going to have to change . . . with all the problems . . . all the government controls."

Lorrimer was originally a pre-med student at Stanford. He then served in the Army Medical Corps; when he returned to civilian life, he decided that he wanted to work in health, but not as a physician. "So, I looked around and hospital management was just coming into being at that time—University of Chicago, Northwestern, Berkeley—they were just starting courses." He then became an administrative resident at the Golden State Hospital, which is in the Western Affiliated Hospital Society system. He worked on the bringing together of the institutions that were to become part of the system in the early 1950s, when the idea of combining resources was extremely radical. Lorrimer has been with the system for over twenty-five years, and is extremely interested in the concepts of control and ownership, believing that it is the power of the boards to "own" a hospital or to influence it that really affects the way that the units work together within a system. He feels that the critical task is to reach the fine line between autonomy of the units and central control.

SUN STATE HEALTH SERVICE

This hospital system grew out of the merger in 1968 of two well-established major hospitals in a southwestern state—Sun State Hospital, a large, acute care facility, and Eastham Hospital, located in a rapidly growing community within the same metropolitan area.

Eastham needed an expanded financial base in order to build a new hospital to replace its outmoded fifty-year-old facility; Sun State needed a broader operational base to utilize its management structure most efficiently and to cultivate referral facilities in the outlying areas to utilize its 715-bed plant downtown.

Within two years, two other community hospitals in the county had been brought into the merging system, along with several rural hospitals in the northern part of the state. Sun State Health Service, a nonprofit corporation, formally incorporated in March, 1970, consists of Sun State Hospital; Desert Hospital and Health Center, a modern 273-bed facility built to replace the original Eastham Hospital; Presbyterian Hospital, a 147-bed hospital; Brookside Hospital, a 62-bed hospital; Mountainside Area Hospital, a 25-bed facility; Sagebrush Clinic, owned by the U.S. Park Service at a national park site, which is in the process of being closed; and Care in the Air, an air ambulance service.

Sun State Health Service is governed by one board of directors and consists of urban, specialty, and teaching hospitals as well as rural community institutions. SSHS is perhaps the best known of the large multihospital systems. It has been studied both formally and informally; the chief executive officer, Trent McLean, has been a national figure since he was named a member of the AHA Board of Trustees and two years later elected to an office. Just as Kaiser became the model of the health maintenance organization, the SSHS quickly became a prototype of the voluntary system that could help reorganize the health delivery system nationally.

McLean reports to a thirty-eight-member board of directors. Seven vice presidents report to McLean, each one holding the title of administrator. Besides the hospitals that are owned by the system, SSHS also operates two institutions under a long-term management contract lease.

There are seventeen competing hospitals in Sun State Hospital's metropolitan area. These include the 560-bed Holy Name Hospital and Medical Center and the 250-bed City Lutheran Hospital. (The latter is owned by St. John's Hospitals and Homes Society.) The area itself is generally considered to be overbedded. As of 1974 none of the seventeen competitors to SSHS had an overall occupancy rate of under 70 percent, and the average daily occupancy rate of the SSHS facilities in 1974 was 64.2 percent.

The CEO

Trent McLean is the chief executive officer of the Sun State Health Service. McLean's background is in the hospital field. He did graduate work in hospital administration and served as administrative resident at the Sun State Hospital in 1953 and 1954. He then became assistant administrator in 1956, administrator four years later, and then president of Sun State Health Service.

McLean has been extremely active nationally in health care. In 1962, early in his career, he was named a member of the American Hospital Association's House of Delegates. He served in the House until 1968, the same year that the Sun State Health Service was formed, when he was named a member of the AHA Board of Trustees. In 1971, he was elected to an AHA office. His work with the AHA led to his role in the Special Committee on the Provision of Health Services headed by Earl Perloff, often called the Perloff Committee. This group came up with the concept of health care corporations, highly integrated hospital systems that would be responsible for providing care in designated areas of the country. Because of McLean's role in national health care and because the system he headed was often referred to as a prime example of a voluntary, not-for-profit innovation that could have significant impact on the delivery of care, the Sun State system received a great deal of attention.

In the early 1970s both the state legislature and a large corporation began programs to control rising health costs. It was not long before the corporation and Sun State Health Service, the first health facility in its area to plan a rate hike, clashed in a public hearing before the local health agency. The corporation embarked on a campaign against SSHS practices that included articles in the company newspaper as well as in local newspapers. Whether or not it was meant to be a personal vendetta between the company's vice president and McLean, the latter viewed it that way. The response to the corporations charges included seven task forces and nine study groups, and demanded a significant amount of time and energy from the CEO and his staff. Perhaps as a result of this process, which did result in some positive changes, Mr. McLean became somewhat publicity shy. He is careful of what he says, and his approach to problems is pragmatic and operational rather than philosophical.

THE METROPOLITAN MEDICAL CENTER

The Metropolitan Medical Center is an excellent example of a carefully executed full corporate merger of three voluntary, nonsectarian, acute general hospitals—former competitors—into a community medical complex of 1,100 beds. It is not only an urban and suburban multiple-hospital system, but also a statewide hospital system, the major medical and health care resource of its state.

Rapidly rising costs, incessant demands for expensive equipment, and the pressing burden of unreimbursed care of indigent patients led, in 1952, to the formation of a Joint Committee. The boards reached a simple agreement to exchange information on wage rates, personnel policies, room charges, and planning for expansion and costly equipment purchases. Unfortunately, the principals were not yet accustomed to thinking cooperatively, and the committee failed to thrive.

It later revived itself and in the early 1960s began meeting regularly. The situation in Metropolitan's home city was unique in that the geographical area was small, it was near medical schools in a neighboring big city, and most important, the three hospitals were remarkably similar: they shared mutual problems, they triplicated attempts to be all things to the same community, they shared their medical staffs, and there were close ties binding many members of the three governing boards.

Metropolitan Medical Center became an entity on November 1, 1965, on the basis that a corporate merger would "best enable those hospitals to provide the highest quality of medical care, strengthen their programs of postgraduate education and avoid costly duplication of facilities."

The city remains closely tied to the vast industrial complexes established long ago in the area. It is similar to many other cities in that the inner city population is only around 80,000, but the county population is an estimated 400,000, and the metropolitan area contains about 510,000 persons. In the decade since the Medical Center was formed, the population has continued to move away from the inner city. This population shift has had considerable impact on strategic planning for the medical center. As pressure grows for health care facilities in the suburbs, heated debate among community groups continues about the likely effect of such facilities on the inner city hospitals. The Metropolitan Facility is gradually being updated and replaced by a 325-bed primary bed care and emergency facility to serve the urban population, while an 800-bed acute care facility on a 200-acre site south of the city is being constructed to serve what has now become the primary area for the Medical Center.

MMC supplies 85 percent of the acute care beds in the city and county, and is the major resource for emergency, outpatient, and rehabilitative treatment for the surrounding area and parts of three neighboring states. The Medical Center is governed by a sixty-seven-member board of trustees, including a number of trustees from the premerger hospitals.

The Medical Center consists of three divisions: the Bayview Division which used to be the Bayview Hospital, and which is being renovated as a more efficient 250-bed community hospital–primary care center, the City Memorial Hospital, known as the Memorial Division, and the Doctors Hospital, known as the Doctors General Division. Substantial construction and renovation has occurred since the merger, including an Ambulatory Service Building and a Coronary Care Unit.

As of 1974, the 1,069 beds provided for 38,599 admissions. The average daily census was 935 and the average occupancy was 88.3 percent. The major problem within this system is financial—MMC has been functioning as an indigent care facility for the state, which has put severe strain on existing resources and has prompted continuous debate with the state about its responsibility to cover reimbursement for charity care. In fiscal 1975–1976, for example, gross charges for services were just over $72 million, with a net gain of $701,000, or just under one percent of gross charges. Because of free care, uncollectable charges, and discounts in government-financed programs, the net income was only $63.8 million. Yet the operating loss was just over $1 million, since operating expenses were kept to a minimum.

The CEO

Byran Miller is the chief executive officer of the Metropolitan Medical Center. With a background in retail management, he decided to go to graduate school after World War II and received his master's degree in hospital administration. He had originally considered medicine and decided against it. His first job in the health area was as administrative resident in an Iowa hospital. From there he went to St. Mark's Hospital in Des Moines, then two years later went to the Queen City Clinic at the age of 31 as chief executive. He stayed for nineteen years.

When he arrived at the Queen City Clinic, it had 320 beds; it now has over 1,000 beds. During that time the clinic grew and matured in every conceivable sense. "We were just getting bigger and bigger and getting into more areas every day—about that time someone asked me if I wanted to come down here, just to look at the setup. I had been interested in mergers because I could see the time coming when small hospitals were not going to make it, and you had to begin putting them together."

Miller feels that his background in retailing made it easy to think in terms of a multiunit hospital system. Yet, when he arrived at Metropolitan, he faced a rather difficult situation; it is still rather problematic to expand into the suburbs "and not make the inner city people feel like we're leaving them behind." Miller was not the prime mover—the person who actually merged the institutions. He took over a number of years after the merger, and is still in the process of stabilizing a complex situation.

Miller is a soft-spoken man who had not taken the position of national leadership of the other CEOs in the study. He sees his main task as developing the people working with him who will some day take over, and one gets the impression that he spends considerable time tending fires at home and relatively little time trying to make a name for himself.

Chapter 6

The Environment

The profiles of the sites presented in the last chapter suggest that the seven multihospital systems have very different characteristics. They are located in varied geographic areas, they were established for unique reasons, and are structured in ways that are specific to their own needs. Yet the data suggest that these seven systems do share a number of critical dimensions. By understanding these shared dimensions—what the systems have in common in terms of their development and their design—both administrators and researchers can have more impact on existing and emerging multihospital systems.

Previous research as well as the literature reviewed in Chapter 4 suggests a number of factors of particular relevance to the development of MHSs. Of these, five appear to have special significance to the environment in which a system operates:

1. The history of collaboration in a region, which tends to facilitate or hinder innovative efforts to combine institutions or portions of institutions.
2. The existence and impact of local pressure groups and organized consumer groups. While regional planning has been a force that medical institutions have had to contend with for a number of years, planning groups now have significant impact on the exis-

tence and growth of these institutions. Community groups can be business groups or community action groups. They can have broad agendas such as the NAACP, which attempts to improve general conditions for the black population, or specific agendas such as a task force which forms to stop the purchase of a particular building and the relocation of its residents.

3. Geographical factors that the systems must take into account. These include the distance between the facilities and the access to each unit, especially the network of highways and the traditional access patterns by which certain patients tend to obtain care at one site rather than at another. While certain aspects of geography are unlikely to change, such as the availability of roads or the topography of the region which might constrain access, it is possible for a system to change its geographic boundaries and to broaden its base of operations so that it begins to provide care in a "new" area, or to avoid expansion in other areas.

4. The competition that traditionally exists in one area among providers that may or may not be evident to consumers. While an increase in the scope of services may be viewed by consumers as a positive action because it is likely to benefit them, the same expansion may be viewed by competitive providers as a serious infringement on their territories.

5. The ability of consumers to pay for their own health care. If, for example, the area has a high per capita income, implying that the average consumer is capable of paying for a portion of his care (catastrophic injury or illness is naturally excluded), then the role of an MHS is likely to be different than in an area where most consumers are unable to contribute. In the first instance, the system can usually depend on internally generated revenues, while in the second the system must develop a far broader financial strategy that includes a high degree of leverage. In addition, the degree of poverty in a given area suggests the kinds of care that patients will need as well as the kinds of professional and unskilled staff that the system will be able to recruit. Consequently the area's per capita income can have significant impact on the development of the system.

While all of these factors are relevant to each system, they vary in their degree of salience. The SSHS, for example, was hindered by the criticism of community groups that were able to exert a great deal of pressure on the system, while in Hillcrest community groups were far less important as a group to contend with. Each system can be described as having a different "profile" in terms of the relative salience of one factor rather than another.

This chapter will be devoted to an exploration of the environment in which each system operates, and will examine some of the ideas presented above.

HISTORY OF COLLABORATION

An appropriate equilibrium must be reached between the external environment and the component parts of the system so that the care of patients can continue with a minimal amount of destructive tension. Thus the factors that affect each system must be understood to judge the appropriateness of the system's responses to these environmental conditions.

There has been a limited tradition of collaboration among American hospitals. Each institution has attempted to exist as if other, comparable institutions did not exist. While at face value this does not seem to be logical behavior, it is in fact more logical to attempt totally autonomous behavior than to admit the availability of limited services. Since collaboration usually implies that, in order to gain something, such as a greater number of patients referred to an oncology service, something else is given up, such as obstetric patients, a collaborative venture suggests limited services. With such a limitation it has traditionally been difficult to raise community funds for the expensive technology that is likely to attract first rate physicians. As funding sources have increasingly come from outside the community, the existence of fragmented services has been viewed as somewhat less of a disadvantage. Certain areas have always been more conducive to collaborative efforts than other areas. What is accepted by planners as well as consumers in one part of the country may still be viewed as a potentially detrimental innovation in another.[1]

In one midwestern city, for example, the concept of collaboration among health institutions is well accepted. Besides the HCH, there are a number of other systems, including Medical Central, which operates four short-term general hospitals in two states. Additionally, Medical Central has affiliate agreements for shared services at thirty-seven other hospitals and nursing homes. Besides HCH and Medical Central there is also the Minnesota Health Center which is an association of four institutions.

Other areas, however, are quite different. In California, Mr. Lorrimer feels that the strong tradition of "rugged individualism" often precludes collaboration. In the East, where the MMC is its principal area provider, there is such a strong feeling of autonomy among the three institutions in question that achieving significant collaboration has been a continuing problem. The situation in Springvale, on the other hand, has been quite different. The SHS was established as a result of an act of the state legislature, and the system grew in response to a changing population and changing needs. Thus the system has not been forced to operate and develop in a climate hostile to collaboration.

This variable can be measured in a number of ways. A spectrum of one to five is useful, one being least conducive to collaboration activity and five most conducive to such ventures. The seven sites would look as follows:[2]

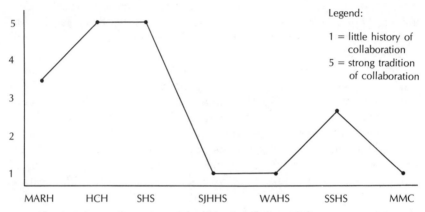

Figure 6.1. History of collaboration.

LOCAL PRESSURE GROUPS AND PLANNING AGENCIES

All the systems studied have been affected by the existence of local groups and planning agencies. The character and activities of such groups have varied considerably, from ethnic populations who have informally tried to inhibit the system's expansion, to organized lobbies of consumers who have effectively stopped further growth. Perhaps the experience of the SSHS and MMC best illustrate the potential impact of local pressure groups on the developing MHS.

Metropolitan Medical Center

When Bryan Miller first came to the Metropolitan Medical Center in 1971, he was in the unenviable position of taking over a recently merged institution which had previously been three separate hospitals, all located in a volatile urban environment. While the MMC feels strong pressure from planning agencies to deliver care efficiently, the urban population, which is now half black, is strongly motivated to encourage the system to remain downtown where it can provide conveniently located care. The two arguments are strong. In the decade since MMC was founded, there has been considerable population growth to the southwest, which has no acute general hospital, and the state planning agencies have made it clear that if the MMC did not address this issue they would have someone else build one. Consequently, the MMC has attempted to meet this need by offering to build a new facility in the southwest area, combining two of the downtown facilities and closing another. While MMC argues that efficient transportation linkages would be provided and that emergency care would continue to be available in the inner city, the black population logically argues that it would be far more difficult to obtain care in such a fragmented system. The inner city population as well as many of the attending physicians would like to see each unit within the system remain a total service facility.

The system's strategy has been to move towards a network of care whereby comprehensive services are available, albeit under two roofs, rather than one. The financial drain of operating the existing facilities with the high level of indigent care has led to significant operating deficits, yet it is easy to understand the antagonism of the urban population who view the possibility of a suburban facility with alarm.[3]

The arguments made by the urban groups that continue to exert pressure on the MMC are certainly rational, as is the argument made by the system itself. The situation is still unsettled, but the process of deciding who to work with in order to make the necessary decisions and how to involve the relevant consumer groups has necessitated constant input about community needs, opinions, and biases, all equally important in a complex urban environment.

Sun State Health Service

A very different kind of community pressure group existed in SSHS's area, where the arguments appear to have been far more inexact and just as detrimental to the development of the system.

A principal objective of McLean's system has been to develop a regional referral center with outreach capabilities. In the process of achieving this objective, the system has successfully surmounted a major problem with a community group: a national corporation with strong local political influence. While a business is seldom viewed as a community pressure group, a private enterprise that is perceived by consumers as being financially strong can very effectively block the expansion or the development of an autonomous hospital or a hospital system.

In the early part of the 1970s, both the state legislature and the corporation became interested in the problem of rising health costs within the state. In 1972, legislation was passed requiring hospitals to seek a review from local and state health agencies for rate increases for major expansion or capital purposes. At the same time, the corporation was conducting a review of hospital costs in an effort to control employee premiums.[4] Consequently, the corporation and Sun State Health Service, the first county health facility with plans to raise rates, clashed in a public hearing before the local health agency in November 1972.

Once the conflict had begun, the hospitals challenged the corporation to debate the issue. The corporation countered by requesting cost and budget information. On the basis of that data, recommendations were made in a study financed by the corporation. The company stated that SSHS's costs could be reduced by more than $5 million per year and that if its recommendations were followed, rate increases would not be needed in 1973 or 1974.

The recommendations were particularly interesting in that many were made entirely from the perspective of a for-profit company that was accustomed to straightforward cost benefit analysis, and used this same approach in assessing whether or not an institution should be merged or whether a specialized service could or could not be justified. Some of the recommendations were certainly warranted and were, in fact, substantiated, while others were refuted; but the conflict serves as a useful illustration of the problems in recommending a straightforward financial approach to the operating and organizational problems of a hospital.

For example, the charge was made that "Sun State should either obtain commitment from local communities to subsidize operating losses at Sun State's four regional hospitals or terminate its operation of them." The system refuted this, stating that a cost reduction and physican recruitment program had begun and that the local communities were being encouraged to absorb operating deficits. It would seem that from the vantage point of the system and from that of the patients served by the system, losses had to be sustained until such a point that the communities could begin to carry them. The corporation found this practice to be highly questionable and countered with the suggestion that the "losing" facility should be closed. SSHS's position was that closing a hospital and curtailing services so drastically was far more serious than closing a plant. While jobs would be lost in both situations for the communities in question, additional risks would exist in prematurely closing a hospital, whatever the operating deficits were, to say nothing of the public outcry that would have ensued after such a decision.[5]

In order to respond to the corporation's charges, and in an effort to involve consumers in the deliberations, seven task forces and nine study groups led by SSHS trustees were established. This unique community effort, which involved 150 private citizens, was aimed at helping SSHS to contain hospital costs and to plot the course of future hospital development. Task force members included homemakers, lawyers, industrial engineers, property management experts, and physicians, among others.

Without doubt, this level of community response was reactive on the part of the system, which did not begin with significant community support. However, many of the groups have stayed on as permanent advisory groups. Undoubtedly the controversy led to a reevaluation of organizational responsibility to curtail costs. As one medical newsletter stated: "The controversy has been painful, but it has rejuvenated the boards of all hospitals and sharpened the thinking of all administrators regarding their responsibility to the public and their own institutions."

And to some extent it also led to short-run cost reductions. For example, Sun State withdrew plans to raise rates in some hospitals and delayed some expansion plans in construction and in medical programs. However, it is still unclear what the long-term effect of the controversy was. According to an official report:

> The chairman of the SSHS board of directors believed that the controversy hurt the image of all the hospitals, particularly that of Sun State, which experienced a drop in usage. Referring to the $2.9 million cutback in SHS operations, he stated, "I think we trimmed a little bit more than the fat because we cut down on much of our capital improvement programs. I don't think it has hurt our programs yet, but if we don't do something [about higher rates] in the next few months, it will start hurting the quality of care."

Whatever the long-term effect is and will be on the delivery of health care in the county as a result of the controversy, it seems clear that the system came to a virtual standstill during this period of time. In an interview, a senior vice president of SSHS stated:

> It took away from my work . . . . I didn't get anything done. That's all we did for a good three years—two and a half years at least. . . . We went on to a series of task forces and study groups . . . . We went on to some-

thing like 18 individual studies with community groups which were pin-pointed by [the corporation]. Some good things came out of that; we set up a very stringent conflict of interest policy concerning the board; we studied this building [corporate headquarters] and found that the $4.50 a square foot we had been paying was probably as cheap as anything we could have gotten . . . but it was a hurdle we had to get over. . . . We were the bad guys because we stand up and we're articulate, we have our slides and charts, we always have to defend ourselves; we had full page ads in the newspaper against us, rebuttals, and rebuttals on the rebuttals. I think it slowed us down considerably in our evolution, in our innovativeness . . . .

There is no reason to think that SSHS could necessarily have fore-seen the impact of this particular environmental demand on the operations of the system, yet it clearly drew a significant amount of time and energy from the system that could have perhaps been spent in more constructive ways. I have recounted this problem with the corporation in some detail because it serves as a particularly good example of the kinds of problems confronting systems and the kinds of problems that can sometimes be avoided by developing an element of community responsiveness before, rather than after, the fact.

This variable can be measured on a spectrum of one to five, five being a system that has had significant demands made upon it by community groups and planning agencies (see Figure 6.2).

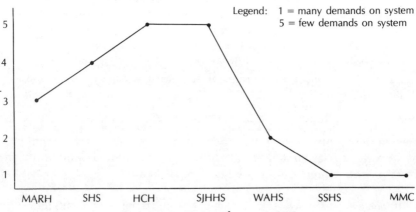

Figure 6.2. Demands on system.

GEOGRAPHICAL FACTORS

Perhaps the most critical geographic factor is the actual distance among the units of a system, and the dispersion of the units within a given region. The STHHS spans an enormous distance, from the southwest to the far north. The MMC, on the other hand, is located within the confines of one major city. While the systems cannot be divided into pure types, they fall into two major categories in terms of their geographical dispersion. The first is the doughnut pattern, where there is one major institution flanked by other institutions that depend on it for referral care and may or may not be smaller. Those systems that began *as* a system have generally grown in such a pattern, including HCH and SHS.[6]

This pattern presupposes vertical integration, with resources being developed on a service area basis with one management assuming responsibility for residents within a given area. The other pattern, which can best be described as a network, is more dispersed. Units are located at randomly spaced intervals from one another and there may or may not be a "prominent" or referral institution. All member institutions usually provide the major services with administrative support and shared services located at another site.

Systems that developed by taking over institutions tend to show this diffused pattern, including SJHHS, WAHS, MMC, and MARH. The Sun State Health Service is somewhat of an exception. It became a system by taking over ongoing institutions, yet there is clearly a dominant institution—Sun State Hospital. These two patterns have significant implications for the development of a system. If, for example, the units are unusually dispersed and there is poor access among them, then a working relationship among the unit heads is unlikely to occur. This is particularly true if they are so dispersed that the relative strength of the environmental factors that affect them is different. The concerns of a rural hospital in Idaho, for example, may be quite different from those of a suburban hospital in Arizona, even though they are both part of the SJHHS.

If, on the other hand, the units are located close to one another, with easy access, then it is difficult to avoid a working relationship; these factors suggest a more participative, decentralized management style. This closeness implies that the boundary scanning function can be done by all of the units and that the information obtained can be regularly supplied to the corporate staff by means of scheduled interactions. To further compound the issue, if the units are close to one another and of approximately equal size and have comparable facili-

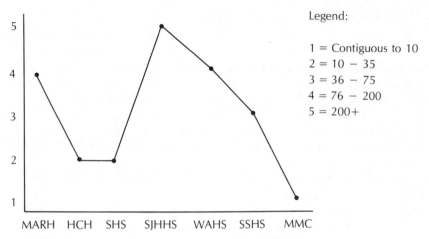

Figure 6.3. Geographic dispersion.

ties, then the issue of effective, long-term collaboration becomes extremely difficult. At the present time, the systems can be described as outlined in Figure 6.3.

In terms of the basic geographical issue of centralization (within 100 miles) versus diffused (outside 100 miles), the profile of the sites would be as shown in the figure.

COMPETITION

Although competition has always existed among health providers, the absence of valid output measures has made it relatively easy to continue operations while remaining both ineffective and inefficient. Reimbursement systems have changed this tradition by setting standards of costs which determine payment, and such measures as PSRO have instituted formal quality control measures. Long before the interest in cost containment, however, hospitals have been interested in maximizing referrals and minimizing the loss of patients to other institutions.

In any one area, a specific set of institutions exists that provides care for the residents of that community. These institutions may be linked to one another in any of a variety of ways, but the purpose of the linkages is to maximize the number of patients that physicians will admit by providing the best possible services. Thus, while the institution prefers to remain autonomous, it often gains more from collaboration than from overt competition. For example, few institutions can offer the patient a full range of oncology care, including preventative education, diagnosis, acute treatment, psychological support, and rehabilitation.

While the patient may enter the system at any one of a number of points, he is likely to need a variety of services, many of which are extremely expensive to provide. For some diseases, such as coronary care, full range care is more widely available. But, in general, institutions must overcome a natural tendency to work autonomously and competitively in order to provide more comprehensive care.[7] The ideal situation for an institution is to maintain control of its patient population by owning, or being able to provide, sufficient resources that a patient[8] need not go elsewhere. However, this ideal situation is difficult to achieve. Patients must frequently look outside for certain services.

The original provider does have certain alternatives in this consumer–provider model. It can use an increasing number of consultative services, thereby increasing the scope of facilities it offers, or it can obtain the funds to hire the necessary expertise. In some cases institutions already possess sophisticated technology and skills that are not efficiently utilized. Therefore, they seek to extend the availability of these services, not because of an innate altruism, but because planning agencies are likely to constrain further development—or force collaboration in a situation where underutilized facilities are evident.

But, in many cases, the original institution becomes a consumer of resources as well as a provider. In order to play both roles with a minimum of destructive tension, it must learn to work collaboratively with other institutions to facilitate access for its own patients who must go elsewhere. Thus the natural fear that collaboration will lead to a loss of patients must be overcome.

While competition is a factor for all the systems studied, it plays a stronger role in certain areas. It must be emphasized that a total lack of competition is just as detrimental to the system's development as a situation where there is constant juggling of patients between consumers and providers. If competition does not exist, then it is difficult for the system to convince the public or the appropriate public agencies that services are being provided cost effectively. As the geographical boundaries of these systems begin to overlap there will be an increasing number of reference points that the systems can use for measurement.

At the present time, SJHHS, WAHS, and SSHS all have units in areas that cross boundaries. Since there is reason to believe that by 1985, 90 percent of the hospitals in the country will be part of an MHS,

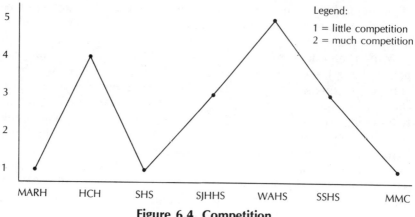

Figure 6.4. Competition.

this issue of competition is likely to become more complex. As expansion becomes more constrained by regulation, competition will have to give way to increased collaboration.

If one were to describe the systems on a spectrum of how competitive the environment is in terms of the existence of comparable facilities, with one equalling little competition and five equalling a high level of competitive institutions, the systems would be represented as shown in Figure 6.4.

SCARCITY OF RESOURCES

The ability of consumers to purchase health care differs significantly both within a system and across systems. In the SJHHS, for example, communities are particularly diverse. In other systems such as SHS, the level of diversity is low since all sites are clustered in or near one city. Because such a broad variation exists, it makes little sense to compute the per capita income in each location and to average the totals. Instead, a rank ordering was developed during the course of interviews. The number one designates that site where more consumers are likely to pay for their own care while the number seven designates that site where the least number of consumers can purchase care:

1. Western Affiliated Hospital Society
2. Sun State Health System
3. Hillcrest Community Hospitals
4. Metropolitan Medical Center

5. Springvale Hospital System
6. St. John's Hospitals and Homes Society
7. Mid-Atlantic Regional Hospitals

The implications of this difference among the sites are interesting. While the importance of diversity within each site cannot be discounted—a range of incomes clearly exists within each area—the health care needs of consumers on the West Coast, for example, are likely to be different from those of consumers in a rural farming state. The first population is more likely to be healthy, and physicians in the area are more likely to show interest in purchasing high technology items than basic clinic furnishings. Financing requirements are also likely to vary: while in a wealthier state revenues can be generated from patient care, rural hospitals in poor areas must be prepared to deliver a greater proportion of free care. In addition, in those areas where resources abound, hospitals can generally service their own debt and obtain outside funding. In areas of scarce resources, however, hospitals are often struggling to become or remain viable and are usually more interested in operating as efficiently as possible than in being able to obtain capital financing.

The level of resource scarcity, then, has implications for the kind and level of services that an MHS provides as well as for its financing requirements.

SUMMARY

The significance of these environmental factors lies in their relative salience and in the salience of one issue rather than another can change dramatically over time. The existence of the factor itself is not as important as the manner in which the system addresses it; this includes diagnosing the actual or potential salience of the factor before it becomes a problem, implying in turn the existence and the ability of a corporate staff able to address such issues.

One can infer from the data that a system faced by a preponderance of negative factors is more likely to require a strong corporate management to deal with such factors and is more likely to experience serious developmental problems than a system faced by a preponderance of positive forces. Consequently, one would expect, for example, that for Metropolitan Medical Center, with:

a low level of collaborative tradition
many demands made on the system by pressure groups

close proximity among units, suggesting the need for a significant level
of cooperation among units
little history of competition with comparable facilities
an average level of available resources

the process of development would be particularly problematic. On the
other hand, Hillcrest Community Hospitals, faced with:

a strong tradition of collaboration
few demands made on the system by pressure groups
fairly close proximity, suggesting a significant but not critical need for
cooperation among units
a significant history of competition among neighboring institutions
a high level of available resources

would be more likely to have a smooth development.

Let us examine the system responses within the framework of these
environmental factors.

NOTES

1. The existence and growth of prepaid group practices is a good example of this.
2. Figure 6.1 and the ones that follow are based on interview data and are clearly
   subjective.
3. It is important to note that the distance between the proposed 800-bed suburban
   facility and the downtown hospital is seven miles, a distance that would be in-
   significant in many systems such as SJHHS. For the MMC this distance has represented a major stumbling block.
4. The campaign was started partially because of the claim that the corporation's
   hospital costs jumped from $1 million in 1966 to $3 million in 1970. A personal
   conversation with an informed participant in February of 1977 yielded the additional
   data that a personal feud existed between Mr. McLean at SSHS and a senior vice
   president at the corporation. This is impossible to verify, and does not alter the effect
   of this outside force on the system.
5. A February 1973 issue of a local newspaper stated: "Hands Off Our Hospital! Enough
   is enough! . . . Your spokesman seems to have solutions to all health care problems.
   One is to close Brookside Hospital. We feel this is just as absurd as if we suggested
   destroying the corporation."
6. Yet SHS and HCH are both in a state of transition: SHS is in the process of developing
   a new site called the Seaver Road Complex, which will be a comprehensive health
   center, while simultaneously closing its downtown acute care hospital. HCH is considering further expansion outside its traditional geographic boundaries.
7. The demands for collaboration will vary as a function of the disease. Chronic dialysis
   for example will necessitate a different pattern of linkages than acute leukemia.
8. The term "patient" is used loosely, for it is the physician rather than the patient who
   makes the decision.

Chapter 7

System Responses

In the previous chapter, the relationship of the seven MHSs to significant environmental factors was discussed. But managers must not only know which factors affect their system and to what degree, they must also be able to respond adequately to any changes in those factors. Responses appear to fall into certain categories:

The ability to deal with planning and community groups in a way that does not allocate an inordinate amount of time to these outside forces to the detriment of ongoing operations.

The ability to finance the system's expansion as well as its operating expenses.

The ability to measure the costs and performance in the individual components of the system. As consumers and planning agencies become increasingly sophisticated about cost containment it becomes more important for the systems to measure and control the performance of their component units.

The ability to publicize the system at the local level, so that existing and potential consumers understand the extent and cost of the facilities available to them, and at the national level, where policies such as P.L. 93–461 encourage collaborative modes.

The ability to establish a corporate staff and board structure adequate to assess the demands of the environment and the needs of each unit.

While each system must address all of the above issues, the time at which each issue is addressed and its relative importance will depend upon the particular environmental pressures that the system faces. For example, legitimizing or "selling" the system has been an important concern in the MMC area, where consumers did not agree with the planned expansion. However, this activity has received far less attention in Hillcrest, where consumers more readily accepted collaborative activities.

MARH, for example, faces quite different environmental demands than MMC. In geographical dispersion, for example, the MMC was rated as a one (contiguous to ten miles) and MARH a four (76 to 200 miles). In its climate for collaboration the MMC was rated a one (little tradition of collaboration) and the MARH a three (significant tradition of collaboration). While these measures are subjective, they do suggest that a system that is geographically centralized and operates in a climate where collaboration is not easily accepted is likely to behave differently than a system that is geographically decentralized and where collaborative efforts are not viewed with alarm.

It might be said that the activities chosen and the emphasis on one activity over another represent an operating strategy for the systems. The concept of a strategy is somewhat novel for hospitals, since it is generally assumed that the objective of all health care institutions is to serve the sick in a given area. It is important, however, to break down this broad altruistic goal into specific tasks that together form the operating strategy for the organization.

Any large organization tends to have a variety of goals. These may range from "being a good place to work" to "being the highest producer in the industry." Thus varied goals may not necessarily be in conflict with one another and may simply represent the varied interests of the people within the organization. However, varied goals can reflect a lack of consensus within the organization about what the long- and short-term goals can and should be. In a complex institution such as a multihospital system, conflict about purpose and goals often arises from the difference in needs and incentives of the major participants: the administration, the trustees, the medical staff, and community groups.[1] As a result of these conflicts, an institution often avoids defining its overall strategy.[2]

It seems clear that a sound strategy for an MHS would achieve adequate congruence between environmental demands and the perceived objectives of the organization. In this chapter, each site will be discussed with specific reference to those five factors that seem to be of particular importance to the development of an MHS. The environmental conditions that each system must address will briefly be summarized, then each site will be separately discussed.

MID-ATLANTIC REGIONAL HOSPITALS

MARH is a predominantly rural system that faces the problem of providing care to an indigent population. The system, which is twenty-five years old, is in an area with historically little collaboration. But like the SJHHS, rural community hospitals find it increasingly difficult to obtain funding and management skills, and consequently collaborate out of necessity.

The system has been developed with the help of community groups that have served as advisory councils. These councils are unique in that the system's corporate headquarters staff has encouraged their establishment in order to increase the communities' involvement with their hospitals. Again, like the SJHHS, the MARH system has not found competition to be important in its development; the rural institutions in question are generally the only providers in a given community.

The Mid-Atlantic Regional Hospitals have a particularly interesting history in that the system was established to provide care for miners and their families. A decade after the hospitals were originally opened, the UMW said that its fund could no longer support four of the five hospitals; the communities would have to take them over within a year, or the facilities would have to close. The problems at the time appeared to stem from a fixed patient base coupled with increased operating costs for the institutions and a decreasing need for coal. Consequently, UMW officials feared, with reason, that the hospital deficits would threaten the fiscal integrity of the UMW fund. However, real community control was impossible, since communities had neither the money nor the management capability to operate the hospitals.

A minister in one of the hospital communities recognized the futility of the situation and appealed to the Board of National Missions of the United Church of Christ. As a result, by October, 1963, the five Mid-Atlantic Regional Hospitals were consolidated under the aegis of a nonprofit, church corporation responsible for operating them. In 1964, five more hospitals joined the system.

Even with a history of critical financial problems, no effort appears to have been made at this time to strengthen the financial base of what was then and continues to be an innovative and truly comprehensive health system. Each hospital has an emergency room and an outpatient clinic, each facility provides home health care services, and there are extended care facilities at four institutions. Yet, the per capita income in this area is so low that the patient population could not pay for their care twelve years ago when the system was founded; they are even less able to pay for it now. Each of the three presidents of the MARH has faced similar problems with reimbursements and indigent care. While the system was run autocratically, continuing the history of absentee direction with most policy decisions being made in Washington by the UMW through its Welfare and Retirement fund, at the local level efforts were made to obtain community support.

Dr. Yellen, the first president of the MARH, established central management offices about seventy miles from the nearest facility. Advisory councils, and later local boards of trustees, were established in each of the ten communities to encourage community involvement. The corporation's objective at the time was to create a sense of interdependency among the units while at the same time assuring central control. While Dr. Yellen did at least attempt to build support for the hospitals at the community level, he did not develop an operating strategy to achieve real decentralization, and the financial problems that have traditionally plagued the system worsened rather than improved.

The second president of MARH, A. C. Swanson, served the system from 1966 to 1973. Under his direction, the system rapidly developed extensive home health care. Again, little attention appears to have been paid either to creating a revenue base with which to fund this valuable activity, or to developing a structure through which a strategy could be implemented. When Dr. Dyer, who had been a board member since the inception of MARH, became president in 1973, the situation was critical and the prognosis poor.

Dr. Dyer has reevaluated the apparent goal of the system—to provide comprehensive care to the rural poor—and believes that if an appropriate strategy cannot be created to fulfill this objective, then the only recourse is to drastically reduce the services provided and, in fact, to risk the total closure of the system. When he arrived at the hospital, Dr. Dyer wanted to address four tasks:

to find the causes of the system's problems
to reorganize the system to be able to fulfill its objectives
to make it cost effective
to make it financially viable in the long run

His approach has been to decentralize the system, emphasizing control from the bottom up rather than centralized at the corporate level. He has established a management information system and relies on only two vice presidents, rather than the five that were there in 1973. Additionally, he had reduced the number of system employees from 3,300 to 500 while at the same time maintaining the same level of comprehensive care. While he feels that he has succeeded in locating the causes of the problem, and has begun to reorganize the system into a workable structure, recent problems have worsened the economic situation. Rather than being able to address the third and fourth tasks—to make the system cost effective and financially viable—his energies have been spent on keeping the system alive, as a result of a number of strikes that seriously depleted the available funds for medical care.

Administrators in each of the ten institutions report to Dr. Dyer, who in turn reports to the thirty-three-member central board. In a further effort to integrate the ten institutions while retaining their autonomy, two members of each advisory council serve on the MARH board. But a workable equilibrium has not been reached for two reasons:

1. Because of the constant financial pressures, the units have never really been *able* to be independent. Health care is considerably more expensive to provide than illness care, since it requires preventive care as well as acute intervention. In addition, the system serves an area that has a high proportion of people unable to pay for care, either "health" or "illness." How is the system to survive? Real autonomy is impossible as long as the financial pressures remain so great that planning at the community level must play a subordinate role to crisis management.
2. Although the aim of the system has been to provide comprehensive care (preventive as well as acute) to those communities, there have never been enough funds available within the communities to pay for it. Consequently, the units have had to subordinate themselves to the overall system in order to continue delivering care.

While Dr. Dyer does appear to address the financial demands of providing comprehensive care, the data suggest that his predecessors never pursued sources of revenue other than the United Mine Workers. As a result, services have been developed with little concern for what was economically feasible. In a sense, the MARH system's current problems can be thought of as microcosms of the problems within the whole health care system: revenue generation has traditionally played a secondary role to the development of services. But it is no longer possible to develop services in a financial vacuum. Issues of capacity, utilization, and reimbursement are as important as issues concerning patient care.

There is no "right" answer to whether a system should insist that its units be financially independent, or simply that the system as a whole be solvent. But whichever choice MARH had made, a more effective boundary scanning function would have shown the dangers of providing extremely costly comprehensive services that the system's units could not support either separately or together without UMW funds.

One would assume that the geographic proximity of the units would have suggested the wisdom of increasing integration among system facilities. But leadership was based in Washington, a situation unique to this system. Perhaps the dependence on external funding discouraged formal or informal cooperation among units in doing organizational or financial planning, or in any attempt to link the two. The strategic development of outreach and comprehensive care, instead of being tied to available funds, was planned in a vacuum.

That leadership changed at critical times increased the lack of congruence between what the system *wanted* to do and what it was able to do. Although MARH's environment was not supportive in the sense that there was little history of collaboration, it was by no means antagonistic. Yet because of poor planning, the leadership was able to make little use of community support. Now, regardless of Dr. Dyer's capability and willingness to diagnose and treat the problem, the strategy of the system must now be radically altered to successfully contain costs. Yet the change required is by no means clear. Reducing internal staff, for example, as a way of containing costs may in the long run be damaging since a lack of corporate staff almost always compromises long range planning. Perhaps a reappraisal of operating and financial strategy would suggest a way to curtail services temporarily, with the intention of expanding them as the level of available revenues increases.

Summary

This system is unusual in that its revenue base has been inconsistent; external funds have usually arrived in time to keep the system functioning, but at inconveniently irregular intervals. Thus, the system was forced to depend upon a kind of deus ex machina to step in to save the system at critical points. Consequently, the system's internal management did not learn to balance a budget, or to plan for gradual expansion and possible contraction of services. The United Mine Workers could have acted to force the system to be more programmatically and fiscally responsible: for example, they could have insisted that funds supplied by the UMW be matched by internally generated revenues, or encouraged the system to formulate and implement a strategy to provide regular revenues.

It is possible that if such fiscal and programmatic responsibility had been encouraged by the UMW, the corporate headquarters in turn might have been able to encourage enough fiscal efficiency in the small community hospitals to allow them to remain self-sufficient. This is in fact what Clarence Coleman has accomplished in the St. John's Hospitals and Homes Society. His goal has not been to encourage collaboration among institutions or to establish expensive and innovative programs, but instead to insure the viability of rural hospitals by instituting control systems and other measures of efficiency.

HILLCREST COMMUNITY HOSPITALS

Hillcrest Community Hospitals, which is twelve years old, is geographically compact, with all units located within a twenty-five-mile radius. It has a long history of collaboration with a number of other cooperative ventures in the same area. Although it has not been significantly impeded by community pressure groups, it has had to deal with competition, since it is only one of a number of groupings in the area. The system is run by Wayne Garrett, who was president of Hillcrest Hospital Association (HHA), a corporation which operated Hillcrest Hospital and a satellite suburban hospital, Hillcrest–Willowdale. In 1973 he became president of Hillcrest Community Hospitals (HCH), a nonprofit holding company established through the consolidation of HHA and another corporation, the Memorial Hospital. This formal consolidation of HCH is more significant than a three-hospital structure would suggest because of the corporation's extensive management contracts and because of Garrett's visibility both as a national leader and as a proponent of the holding company concept.

A holding company in health care would be similar to one in banking, where one company with a central corporate office, board, and management has ownership control over one or more member banks, each operated by its own board of local civic and business leaders. A key characteristic of a holding company is that when it purchases a corporation, it absorbs all of the corporation's property, assets, and income as well as debts, liabilities, and obligations. With this structure, Garrett believes that the component parts of a health care system can be responsive to community needs as well as efficiently managed.

Although HCH's corporate strategy has evolved significantly since 1952, Hillcrest has been a religious-based hospital since it was founded in 1905 by a group of Finnish ministers, a fact that is still important in determining operational and financial strategy.

When Garrett was appointed administrator, Hillcrest was a single hospital of 172 beds operating at a deficit. By 1954 Garrett had turned the hospital around financially, and between 1952 and 1963 he also installed the city's first private hospital psychiatric unit. During these early years, Garrett felt that the critical tasks were to build competent boards, to improve the self-image of the management staff at the hospital, to build up enthusiasm for the hospital internally and externally, and to assemble a senior management group. At the same time, plans were being made to build a satellite, Hillcrest–Willowdale, to provide services to the southwestern suburbs.

The proposals for Hillcrest–Willowdale faced as little opposition as did the first satellite hospital in the SHS. And in fact, one would expect little conflict or tension when a system expands not by co-opting another institution, but by building in response to changing needs.

"We could see a void in South Hillcrest," said Mr. Bergman, a trustee since 1938 and chairman of the board of New World Life Insurance Company, looking back over the years.

> The Milton Corporation was developing this property to be the first major suburban regional shopping center in the upper Midwest. Milton bought half their land from me. I always wanted to see some of that property go to the hospital and I wanted Milton to give Hillcrest 25 acres. We compromised at 15. We were fortunate to have Wayne as Administrator. He could see the opportunity as much as I could and we encouraged each other.

The opening of Hillcrest–Willowdale also represented the beginning of a new financial strategy. During Hillcrest–Willowdale's early development, Hillcrest Hospital had provided financing, medical staff, personnel, and experience, while enduring criticism from urban residents for giving in to the pressure of suburbanization. Hillcrest–Willowdale, once financially sound, contributed its income after expenses to defraying the high cost of service at Hillcrest Hospital, located in a declining area. Any facilities and service lacking at Hillcrest–Willowdale were provided to Willowdale patients at Hillcrest by transporting them to the in-town hospital at hospital expense.

With the Hillcrest Affiliate Program, begun in 1970, four hospitals agreed to share with Hillcrest such services as data processing, materials management, and stores management. In order to encourage these affiliative agreements, Garrett stressed that community hospitals had a great deal in common and that agreements to share a variety of services would not lead to a loss of patients for physicians in the outlying communities. He urged that the agreements be seen as a consultation with peers—as a tie, not a takeover.

This pattern of growth continued, and led to a consolidation agreement with the Memorial Hospital in 1972. This affiliation is a particularly interesting illustration of Hillcrest's strategy, in that the eighty-five-year old institution located in a deteriorating downtown area and faced with rising costs and a declining census, chose between the proposals of Crosley–Riverside (who suggested a corporate merger) and Hillcrest (who suggested Memorial be adopted into a holding company).

Garrett suggested that Memorial continue to have its own board of trustees and its own medical staff, as well as the distinctive programs that identified the hospital within its community. At the same time, Memorial would become part of the larger Hillcrest structure and receive advice and financial support. The amount of representation Memorial would have on the Hillcrest Hospital Association (the corporate) Board would be in proportion to the ratio of their respective assets.[3]

Although the Memorial staff had stronger ties with Crosley Hospital than with either of the Hillcrest Hospitals, the medical staff and the board of trustees voted strongly for the Hillcrest proposal. Garrett felt that the vote represented an important acceptance of the holding company concept: "That was a dramatic and critical meeting for us . . . if the physicians voted in favor of the Crosley–Riverside proposal, our holding company concept would have been just a piece of paper." Memorial's present administrator, Wallace J. Mason, explained why the board opted for HCH:

> We could only maintain our role by being part of the cash flow of a larger organization. The Board felt that the philosophy of a multihospital corporation—the concept of continued identity, a separate medical staff, a fair amount of autonomy, a separate board—was more consistent with Memorial's philosophy than a merger.

It would seem then that Memorial is in a stronger position in HCH than Hillcrest–Willowdale, only because it has a separate corporate identity and has retained its own board while Hillcrest–Willowdale was created as and remains a satellite unit. In addition, Garrett appointed the administrator of Memorial, indicating the hospital has considerably less autonomy than appearances might suggest, although an effort has to be made to retain at least symbolic autonomy. Garrett said about this appointment:

> I chose Wally Mason from outside Hillcrest because of the requirement of the position. This was a delicate time and Memorial needed strong leadership. We needed maturity and experience and I needed someone to fit into that environment. The men on my staff either didn't want to, or weren't able to, go over there. For Don and his adminstrators, it would be a step down. If Bob or Ted had wanted to go over there, the presence of a Hillcrest man would make the consolidation look like a takeover. We were fearful of that sort of analysis. Any other logical person over here wasn't Lutheran. At Memorial, it was essential that the new administrator be Lutheran.[8]

It would seem that, for better or worse, Memorial is in fact only marginally more autonomous than Hillcrest–Willowdale, in spite of a declared intention to protect its independence.

When Memorial became part of HCH in 1973 its assets were $6.5 million. The hospital has been operated profitably ever since, and today assets exceed $7.5 million. The same considerations—financial survival and stability—brought Harbridge Community Hospital, north of the city, to HCH. Harbridge, however, chose a different level of participation; at present, it is the only facility with a management contract with HCH, although it is requesting ownership.

When Harbridge first considered joining HCH, it faced serious problems. Its expenditures surpassed income, and the chairman of the board reputedly had not spoken to the medical staff chief in more than three months. Negotiations resulted in a three-year management contract that allows Harbridge to draw upon Hillcrest's managerial expertise. HCH selects and pays Harbridge's administrator and is responsible for the total hospital operation—daily operations, long-range planning, medical staff, and community and third-party coordination. This 39-bed institution made $68,000 in 1976 and, more importantly, the community is solidly behind the hospital. As Garrett said, "As the economic pressures increase in the health field, our holding company would be one consideration for these boards to look at . . . to have management contract or ownership. It gives a local hospital the option of being a freestanding institution."

In an area that is as "affiliation oriented" as Hillcrest, community institutions had considerable choice when they came to HCH. It appears they were attracted to the operating and financial strategy of the system, or at least to those parts that were visible.

After establishing ties with Memorial and Harbridge, Hillcrest devised a new strategy, one that is still operative today. Garrett felt that, in addition to directly providing services, Hillcrest ought to encourage others to improve their health delivery throughout the state. As part of this strategy, Garrett mobilized new and existing facilities and programs to provide health care to the residents of a new housing project in the city. So, while HCH has grown in the past by collaborating with hospitals that share its religious orientation and are within 300 miles, Garrett now considers these factors considerably less important as he plans future growth.

Between 1952 and 1974, his strategy was to expand through a holding company concept. He achieved his objectives of building the reputation of the hospitals and establishing a strong board and a competent management group, all with a central administration that remained remarkably unchanged.

Like all the hospital systems studied, the Hillcrest Hospitals' management system was a combination of centralized and decentralized functions. As president of the Hillcrest Hospital Association, Garrett was responsible for implementing policy and for operations in both hospitals. As CEO of the holding company, he was responsible to the HCH Board and had general supervision, direction, and management control of the business and of all other officers of both HCH and its constituent corporations. Thus, his responsibilities extended over Hillcrest, Hillcrest–Willowdale, and the Central Division, which served these units as well as the four affiliated hospitals and Memorial.

Garrett delegated most of these responsibilities to the hospital administrators—Theodore Law, Robert Brown, and Wallace Mason—and to Glenn Garman, assistant administrator in charge of the Affiliate Division. While Brown and Law both developed their careers in the Hillcrest system, Mason was new to Hillcrest and somewhat older than the other two men. Although some major functions, such as fiscal management, were centralized at one hospital for the others, some functions continued to exist as separate departments.

Although the organizational chart during these years suggests Law and Brown had considerable authority, it seems clear that significant decisions were made by Garrett in conjunction with Mr. Bergman, the very powerful board member who until recently had considerable power within the system. As long as the system consisted of only two hospitals, the structure was adequate, but as growth continued, strains became apparent.

Garrett felt that it was impossible to change the structure in any significant way as long as "Berg" remained a critical force. Under Bergman's influence, board meetings were held only four times a year, for one hour. One infers from conversations with Garrett that although the board consisted of respected and competent community leaders, there was little policymaking, or even information sharing, at its meetings. Committees were not looked upon favorably by Mr. Bergman, and it seems clear in retrospect that the two administrators in the second tier of management came to feel they had little power, with no immediate prospect of getting more.

This stress within the system led to a reevaluation of the structure and of the overall strategy and eventually to a reorganization. During the year (1977) that "Berg" was away, Garrett formed a committee of five senior vice presidents of major corporations in the area to evaluate the system and to recommend structural changes that could help achieve the high level of growth the system sought. This move not only reaffirmed Garrett's own power and reduced Bergman's, it also resulted in the formation of two vice presidencies for Law and Brown, with considerable power delegated to both by Garrett.

Change, then, has been significant. The strategy now emphasizes growth—perhaps in the form of an affiliation with a 450-bed hospital in a neighboring city and with a 480-bed out of state. Senior management has been decentralized, with Garrett more of an "outside" leader and less an inside manager. These changes are no easier to adapt to than they are to formulate. Garrett says, for example, that he used to work with the medical staff closely, and knew every single decision that was being made. Now he is suddenly aware that the same physician who used to come into his office is going to Brown or Law; he was troubled until he realized that "this is what delegation is all about."

Garrett believes that the objective of the system is to be responsive to local needs by retaining local boards of trustees, while providing an enhanced capital base, superior management, and central services.

Summary

The HCH is situated in an area that encourages collaboration. Its growth has been in two directions: gradually building a system response to community needs and demographic changes, and developing a business that provides management contracts to a wide variety of institutions. The holding company concept is at the core of its management philosophy, and Garrett has spent a significant portion of his time championing this idea both regionally and nationally.

Originally, internal growth was closely managed by a subset of the board and by Garrett. As the system expanded, it became clear that its highly capable management staff was being underutilized. This problem appears to have been corrected in the course of a recent reorganization, and the system now seems in a good position to realize its ambitious plans. Thus the level of congruence between environmental characteristics and HCH's response continues to be high.

THE SPRINGVALE HOSPITAL SYSTEM

The Springvale Hospital System (SHS), which is twenty-four years old, began as a system. Although it is difficult to assess what the history of collaboration is in the area outside of this system, it can be assumed that it is no greater than in the other six sites.

The units of the SHS are located close to one another; they can be reached in a thirty-minute drive from downtown Springvale. Community groups have played an important role in the development of this system. Input from such groups has been used both for long-range planning and as a mechanism to involve patients and potential patients. Since the system began as an act of the legislature, the role of state planning agencies in the development of this system has been viewed as less "antagonistic" than in the other sites.

Competition is not a strong environmental force in the SHS area. Expansion came about as a result of demographic need and, while other providers do exist, the system works with them in developing its own long-range plans. Because the SHS began as a system, it is unique in never having had to face the problem of integrating autonomous units. The system, which now consists of nine facilities, has strong central management and three divisions, each managed by an administrator. It was created by an act of the 1947 state General Assembly, which established the authority for a hospital system serving the county. This act also provided for an independent and self-perpetuating board of trustees which would govern and operate the Springvale General Hospital as a community-oriented, nonprofit, voluntary institution for the benefit of all citizens of Springvale County. But five years later, another hospital was built with twenty-seven beds twelve miles northeast of the city's center. This marked the beginning of what has been continuous system expansion in response to a growing and changing population.

Thus, the SHS was spared many of the development problems faced by the other systems. The relationship of the units to one another has never been antagonistic. Each was built to implement the concept of a comprehensive system of care and was planned in response to a specific need. Consequently, the tension that existed in the other systems between autonomy and interdependence is minimized in the SHS. The system is organized as shown in Figure 7.1.

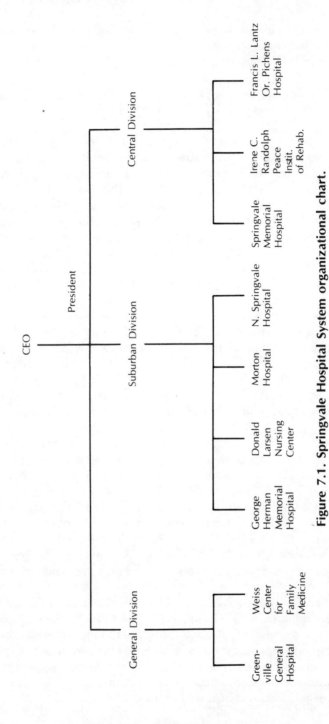

Figure 7.1. Springvale Hospital System organizational chart.

CEO

President

General Division

Suburban Division

Central Division

Greenville General Hospital

Weiss Center for Family Medicine

George Herman Memorial Hospital

Donald Larsen Nursing Center

Morton Hospital

N. Springvale Hospital

Springvale Memorial Hospital

Irene C. Randolph Peace Instit. of Rehab.

Francis L. Lantz Or. Pichens Hospital

These facilities range from acute, general hospitals to long-term rehabilitative and psychiatric institutions. The office of the chief executive officer, Craig Gardner, is located in the center of the system, within a thirty minute drive to any of the units. Gardner reports directly to the board of trustees and is responsible for planning and external relations. Mr. Fisher,[4] the chief operating officer, reports to Mr. Gardner and is responsible for the three divisions as well as for support services. Again, because of the unique beginning of this system, the medical staff is noninstitutional; physicians work within clinical departments but freely cross institutional lines. Although each of the nine units is weak in relation to the system as a whole, they are apparently as strong as they need to be to deliver the most comprehensive and widely used health care in the area. No facility is in a subordinate position to the others, and there appears to be little tension within the system regarding autonomy and interdependence.

The SHS originally emphasized clinically and geographically decentralized service and was vertically organized to address all health care needs in a given geographic area. The emphasis now is on working closely with the communities to become more responsive and to give special attention to the problems of the aged.

> We're much more interested now in the growth and development of concepts as opposed to the growth and development simply of hospitals and beds and doctors. Diagnosing and treating acute illness is very exciting to a lot of people, but it doesn't necessarily meet community needs. Every success we have in the acute phase of illness leaves a residue of chronic illness and now we have to deal with this.

Again, on the topic of the system's evolution, Garner said:

> At the board level we have to change our community relations committee from working on the image of the hospital to working on community activities, to being concerned with providing community health and determining the mission of the hospital. At the administrative level we're trying to deal with all of the illness and disability oriented groups in the community, this tremendous multiplicity of agencies that have no real roots except in the people that have those disabilities, and give them roots at the hospital level, without forcing the hospital on them—give them a place where they can be comfortable, come in with their problems and have their meetings.

Gardner sees this as a move from regarding the hospital as an institution that provides services to a traditional population, to one with a mission to improve the quality of life for all people within the county, including those not accustomed to using hospitals at all.

In order to do this, SHS relies heavily on the fifteen-member advisory councils, representing the county's four service areas, to link it to its communities. They meet monthly, are briefed on system plans, and are urged to advise hospital leadership concerning needs and problems requiring attention in their areas. The councils have participated in naming a new hospital, assisting in the creation of an auxiliary for the new hospital (at Endicott), a survey of health care needs, development of a "no smoking" policy in each hospital, and recruiting physicians.

What these advisory councils actually accomplish is probably less important than the fact that they exist. In addition to symbolizing SHS's concern for community interests, the councils allow SHS to anticipate potentially disruptive community encroachment by continually scanning its boundaries to diagnose changes in the environment that may create problems.

Summary

SHS is unique among the seven systems studied in having begun its corporate existence *as* a system, by state mandate. Consequently, the issue of collaborative environment has not been important. Perhaps because executive energies did not have to be spent establishing relationships with potential members, they appear to have been spent establishing liaisons with community groups that have participated significantly in the planning of the system.

In addition, the system is unique in having addressed the issue of management succession. Gardner has traditionally played the role of leader who scans the environment and links the system to the outside. There is also an internal leader, primarily concerned with system affairs.

In summary, the fit between the environment and the system appears to be excellent in the SHS. Yet it must be remembered that the environment has been unusually accepting of such a venture, and that the system, having been mandated by the state government, has needed little effort to attain legitimacy.

WESTERN AFFILIATED HOSPITAL SOCIETY

Unlike the SHS, the Western Affiliated Society of Southern California is not geographically compact. Its facilities spread over 150 miles, and the system is marked by a spirit of individualism that encourages autonomy and discourages collaboration.

WAHS's development has been influenced by community groups, but the growth of the system as a whole has not been impeded by organized efforts.

Competition is a significant factor; the area is clearly overbedded, and among the several other providers, some are, like WAHS, grouped in a system.

Jesse Lorrimer, the director of WAHS, did not initially define the direction or extent of corporate growth. As a result, several mistakes were made early in the system's life. But Lorrimer believes WAHS has profited from its mistakes, having learned the need to define its own goals and assess environmental forces *before* deciding to expand operations.

Two examples of early errors were the decisions to purchase Colchester and Underhill Hospitals. Colchester, a small community hospital of 130 beds handling 24,000 emergency patients yearly,[5] was located in a community that could not pay for its own care. The hospital proved to be "tough to keep alive." Lorrimer describes Underhill Hospital, purchased subsequently, as their only failure. A group of local residents had secured a Hill–Burton grant to build the hospital, but lacked the management expertise to plan and operate it. Therefore, as part of the purchase agreement, WAHS was to manage the hospital. Underhill, located in a wealthy community of retirees, was to raise $3,000,000 for the project. However, the funds were not raised and the Underhill board wanted to remain closely involved with day-to-day operations, in spite of the management agreement they had signed. It became clear to Lorrimer that the only way to salvage the situation was for WAHS to control the board of directors. This was unacceptable to the community and the arrangement between WAHS and the community came to an end one month before the hospital was due to open.

These early mistakes led Lorrimer to delineate more clearly his own role within the evolving system. He decided his first task was to build a management staff and a central headquarters. During this first stage he moved his office away from the main hospital and into a new headquarters. He said in an interview,

> My position became very lonely. I'm basically a hospital administrator and I love being one. I'm the kind of person who likes to be very close to what's going on. I like being with the nurses, the doctors, touring the hospital in the morning and evening, and telling our administrative people to get out on the floor. When I first became president I moved across the street to a medical building because I knew people would keep

running to me if I didn't move, and it was really very lonely. But quickly I began filling up my time, devising our central organization.

His next task was to establish a structure that could sustain growth while remaining flexible. Lorrimer feels that his principal task now is to legitimize that structure sufficiently to sustain the confidence of committee and board members in the event of a crisis.

In revamping WAHS's structure, Lorrimer formed a profitmaking subsidiary called California Health Management Services, Inc., with two goals in mind. First, he felt that several institutions that WAHS might profitably link up with would respond more favorably to overtures from an organization without any religious ties. Secondly, he believed that the most effective way to market their services as management consultants was through a profitmaking subsidiary.

The structure that has evolved for WAHS, Lorrimer feels, has the benefits of a community hospital but can still compete profitably with other management and shared service corporations.

Thus, Lorrimer has devised and implemented a stragegy which has made WAHS financially successful as well as effective, and has enabled the system to adapt to environmental pressures by developing other revenue bases in addition to the gross revenues of its not-for-profit institutions. Lorrimer's system is characterized by a depth of second-line managers and an innovative approach less concerned with how things "should be done" than with how they "might be done" to work best for WAHS. For example, while Lorrimer feels that *in general* the easiest board structure for an MHS is one board owning a number of hospitals, such as the Sun State Health Service model, he himself has placed

an administrator in each hospital, which is what McLean has as well, but my administrators report to their own boards, so they end up with two bosses, which is bad management . . . but it works. Knowing the climate here, I felt that the best way to go was a sort of horizontal management thing, with interlocking boards, with the boards understanding that their administrator was reporting to me as well as to them. The reason it works is that the Board at the individual hospital makes the political decisions and even if I don't agree with it, the administrator and I have to follow it. It isn't very often, though, that I don't agree.

In 1975, when WAHS announced the formation of California Health Management Services, all of the corporation's central service functions were shifted into the subsidiary. At approximately the same time, all of the hospital operations and management relationships were spun off into a nonprofit corporation called West Coast Health Management Cooperative.

In redefining WAHS's goals, it appears that Lorrimer considered two interrelated factors in the environment to be paramount: the communities' general emphasis on local control, and consumers' suspicion of health care delivered by an "outside" agent. Said Lorrimer, "I think you can only have good quality medical care and do the things you want to do in the future if there is local control, and I've always felt that our role was to bring this about. . . ."

His strategy for growth takes both factors into account, as well as the fact that the area is generally agreed to be overbedded. Lorrimer believes that the system must grow by responding to requests of viable institutions willing to trade their autonomy for the management skills and capabilities of a larger system, rather than by purchasing small, underutilized hospitals.

Geography is also a factor in Mr. Lorrimer's decisions:

> We've been trying to get together with the hospitals that are located in the communities we are located in. For example, in Bella Vista, there is a large, good Catholic hospital, St. John's, and we should be working with them because they are only a mile from us.

Summary

The WAHS was an early multihospital system, operating in an area that has traditionally been overbedded and consequently highly competitive. There appears to have been early conflict between the system's desire to secure control in all management agreements, and the communities' desire to retain autonomy. Since that time, the system has retained its important place among not-for-profit multifacility systems, and has become a pioneer in establishing for-profit subsidiaries.

WAHS's overall operating strategy appears to be well balanced. The system is financially sound, and has a competent corporate staff that allows the CEO to spend considerable time outside its geographic boundaries legitimizing its role. It has also developed a mixed and consequently more dependable revenue base by means of its for-profit subsidiaries. The structure of the organization, with its separate boards, emphasis on local control, and a modified matrix structure whereby each administrator reports both to his own board and to the society, appears to be responsive to the environmental characteristics of the area.

ST. JOHN'S HOSPITALS AND
HOMES SOCIETY

The St. John's Hospitals and Homes Society (SJHHS) was begun in 1938 to "provide health care wherever it was needed." The system that resulted is unique, in being the most decentralized geographically of all the systems under consideration. While it is headquartered in the upper Midwest, it can boast ninety institutions in thirteen states, more than any other MHS in existence. Units are small, rural health providers sharing a number of cultural and demographic similarities that form an important bond. While there necessarily could not be a history of collaboration for so many different units in such a variety of locations, collaboration has been enforced by the inability of the individual institutions to obtain adequate financing and sufficient management expertise.

SJHHS has not been particularly affected by strong community groups or planning agencies. In fact, it would appear that the influence of planning agencies would have been felt far more strongly if the financially unsound institutions had remained autonomous. It has not had to be significantly concerned with competition, since each unit is usually the only hospital in a given community. This situation is changing, however, as the environments of the systems begin to overlap.

The SJHHS is operated by Clarence Coleman, relying on six corporate officers to review the activities of all member units, each of which is managed by a "superintendent." The system was established as a result of financial pressures, which came to a head in 1929 when many of the small hospitals serving western and midwestern rural communities were no longer financially viable. Given the low wages that hospitals were able to pay, it was difficult to find adequate administrative skills. As Coleman wrote in a journal article, "The job of administration was often relegated to community members who provided leadership on a part-time, voluntary basis." One answer was to centralize management branching decisions down into programmable components that could be handled in precisely the same way in all the units. Not all of the units are owned by the society; twenty-nine are owned and sixty-one are leased, but all the facilities are managed as if they were owned.

There is strong management control over each institution; the society assumes complete control and complete fiscal and operational responsibility. The units are integrated by a complex management information system that provides daily operating data from each institution. There is, however, little communication among the units, in part because of the geographical distance between them, ranging from eighty to several thousand miles, in part because the system was never intended to provide it. There does not seem to be significant tension between the units and central headquarters: the society comes into an area at the community's request,[6] and although some attempt is made to retain a focus on community care, most local residents appear to recognize that by agreeing to assume a unit's financial problems, the society earns the right to control its operations. And, in fact, the society's domination has saved many rural communities from tremendous medical hardships.

Although Coleman is in the process of establishing regional offices in an effort to decrease travel time and expenses,[7] it appears that he is in control of hiring decisions at all but the lowest level and that he makes most operational decisions. This highly centralized structure is necessitated by the extreme geographic decentralization of the system: in order to respond effectively to changes in ninety complex and dispersed units, information must be fed back quickly to the central authority ultimately empowered to act. The management information system that Coleman has designed effectively accomplishes this.

However, in spite of the units' geographical separation, they share two characteristics: they are all predominantly rural, and they all joined the system primarily for financial reasons. The latter fact has greatly influenced the system's strategy. Coleman feels strongly that each institution should be strong enough financially to secure credit on its own, although, in fact, it is the system as a whole that borrows. Today, the system has a $14 million line of credit, and Coleman is beginning to put less emphasis on capital structure. He notes that the last time the system sold a bond issue, it took only a day and a half to do so, and that his time is now being spent on "melding the tones so that you don't hear one too loudly"—and "one" in this case is the financial strategy.

The society has undertaken a significant number of major construction projects to meet the environmental demands of the sixty-five communities it serves. In Alaska, for example, services have grown to meet the increased demands created by the Trans-Alaskan pipeline. In 1976 and 1977, projects worth $46 million have been completed, ranging from new hospitals to dormitories. Communities are encouraged to raise funds for projects themselves. In another state, construction funds for a nursing home addition were raised by a countywide sales tax increase.

Summary

The SJHHS is unique in that it spans thirteen states and sixty-five communities. From its inception the system has had a clear mission: to allow member units to continue providing care for their communities by taking advantage of the management skills and coordinated services that the system could offer. Consequently, little attention has been paid to integrating the member units beyond the formal multi-institutional system. It would be both extremely difficult to do so because of the system's size, and unnecessary in light of the needs of member units. Similarly, little attention has been paid to building relationships with local community pressure groups. The society is always asked to take over the management of an institution, and the communities appear to recognize that without such management many of these units could not exist. The primary effort within this system has been to ensure sufficient operating revenue for expansion and to control operating expenses. This effort has largely been orchestrated by one person, Clarence Coleman, with the help of a small corporate staff. The question of successor has not been addressed. Coleman is fairly young, in good health, and appears to be able both physically and psychologically to travel a great deal. Thus there seems to be sufficient congruence in this system between the characteristics of the environment and the responses of the organization. It remains to be seen, however, how much of this congruence is dependent on this particular CEO and how much is built into the system.

SUN STATE HEALTH SERVICE

The Sun State Health Service (SSHS) appears to be less compact geographically than it actually is: while the units are spread over a 180-mile radius, the three largest units are located within a 10-mile area.

There is little history of collaboration in this region. But again, in a primarily rural area (outside the central city) it is difficult for general community hospitals to exist without entering into some kind of collaborative arrangement.

Community groups have exerted a profound pressure on the development of SSHS. Although competition has traditionally played a minor role, it is gradually becoming more of a factor, with seventeen potentially competitive institutions now existing in the area.

There are a number of similarities in the early growth of the WAHS and the SSHS. In both of these sites, the CEO initially encouraged rapid growth without sufficiently addressing the development of a structure that could support this growth. In the case of the WAHS this pattern of early growth, which was not always successful, led to a reappraisal of short- and long-term goals. In the case of SSHS a number of errors were made as the system developed, and these earlier errors have resulted in a more capable and probably more efficient system.

Sun State Health Service, Inc., was created during the period from August 1968 to October 1969 by the merger, purchase, and lease of one urban, three suburban, and four rural hospitals. Ninety-two percent of the beds and 95.2 percent of employees are located within the home county, and 70 percent of the population of the county lives in the central city; thus, the system is quite centralized geographically. Although the SSHS is still changing, its initial formation was rapid, extending over only eighteen months. It is perhaps a result of its quick organization that SSHS appears not to have planned its subsequent growth to meet clear corporate objectives.

Development, at least during the early stage, appears to have been random, with opportunities seized as they presented themselves. The system did have goals that are articulated in a number of planning documents, including the *Outline of Health Services* published by the SSHS Office of Planning. The goals outlined were as follows:

> Sun State Health Service exists to improve the level of health in the communities it serves through the development and maintenance of an organized system, providing or participating in the provision of health care services which are comprehensive in scope, reasonably available, high in quality, reasonable in cost, and in keeping with human dignity and community need.

While intrahospital and interhospital services were planned to be coordinated and complementary in order to encourage referral patterns wherever possible, there is no evidence that the issue of how or whether to achieve interdependence was ever addressed. For example:

Were the units to be strong or weak in relation to corporate headquarters?

How much and what kind of information exchange was necessary among the various units?

What was the ideal level of corporate staff in relation to the existing staff within each unit?

Consequently, the lack of clearly defined goals appears to have led to an initially ineffective organizational structure that placed the fragile system in a vulnerable position. McLean has spent little time assessing the peculiarities of his own environment, perhaps because he felt that he knew all there was to know from his more than two decades of experience as a manager at Sun State Hospital. Although this experience no doubt was helpful, there is little evidence to suggest that he understood the political and functional problems facing a *system*; in fact, his perspective was somewhat parochial and idealistic. Over the years the Sun State Hospital had answered many requests from neighboring hospitals for consultation and help. Relationships that developed during these interchanges led to the hospitals' contacting Sun State to suggest a possible merger, and later to the smooth implementation of the merger itself during the transition periods. Yet because McLean never articulated a set of goals more specific than the general ones cited above, member hospitals had little information about expectations or measures of effectiveness.

Most of the hospitals that approached SSHS about a merger did so because of financial problems. The experience of Presbyterian Hospital is illustrative, although perhaps too extreme to be typical. Presbyterian was founded in the late 1950s by a local contractor and land developer. The hospital was in serious financial difficulty almost from the beginning. First, it was necessary to sell an additional $400,000 in bonds in order to complete the project. Patient revenues were inadequate to operate the hospital and pay the interest on the bonds. Then the hospital went through a series of bankruptcy proceedings, lost a securities fraud suit, and suffered other court action before it was placed under federal court supervision in 1964. Between 1964 and 1967, various trustees and administrators were appointed to manage the hospital in the hope of maintaining its solvency. Slowly, the financial position of the hospital began to improve. In 1968, an out-of-state proprietary corporation that already had a chain of hospitals attempted to purchase Presbyterian. A number of citizens and the county Health Planning Council were concerned because they believed that the hospital should be locally owned and controlled. Several other city hospitals were approached before Sun State purchased Presbyterian in 1968. Since the purchase, Presbyterian has prospered; both its admissions rate and its occupancy rate are at a ten-year high, and plans have been made to increase facilities.

The reasons for this improvement are complex: Figure 7.2 shows the organizational structure for Presbyterian at the time of purchase in September 1968, with an assistant and an associate administrator as well as eight department heads reporting to the administrator. Beginning in 1969, with the emergence of a corporate form of organization, an executive vice president was named adminstrator of Presbyterian with two executive directors, the head of personnel, and the head of public relations reporting to him, thus reducing his span of control to four. (See Figure 7.3.) By 1974, the executive vice president's title had been changed to vice president, and two assistant administrators re-

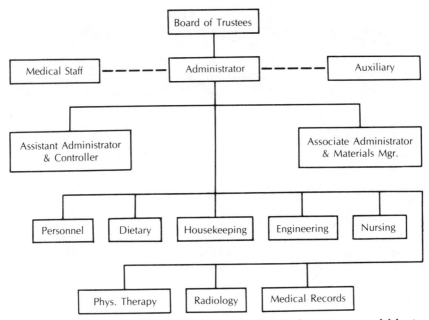

Figure 7.2. Presbyterian Hospital organizational chart (pre-acquisition).

ported to him. In addition he had direct functional responsibility for six departments—personnel, business office, volunteers, public relations, administrative offices, and admitting. (See Figure 7.4.) His span of control increased to eight as a result of his taking on these additional departments.

These changes in reporting relationships reflected a goal of SSHS to eliminate duplicated effort among the hospitals as well as to provide institutional and management services of a higher quality than the hospitals could provide for themselves. The objectives of SSHS at this time were adequately summarized in an AHA report:

SSHS sought to convince the individual hospitals that by consolidating some activities with the other hospitals they would be able to take advantage of certain economics of scale and levels of specialization which would be impossible if each hospital were to act independently. However, each hospital would lose some of its autonomy and flexibility if it agreed to participate since central planning and standard procedures would be required.

SSHS had the problem of designing an efficient system which could take advantage of economies of scale (for example, through purchasing large lot sizes) and increased specialization (for example, employing experts and specialists and purchasing special purpose equipment which smaller hospitals could not justify economically) without drastically disrupting the autonomy of the individual hospitals. SSHS was also under pressure to provide quality services at competitive prices because, if the hospitals found themselves charged with sharply rising costs for sustaining staff services, they would likely question the value of these services. In addition, if the hospitals believed that the services were ineffective, that attention to their particular needs was lacking, or that reports required for their operation lagged, pressures to decentralize would arise.

Hospital personnel increased from 2,510 in 1968 to a high of 3,342 in 1971. However, as a result of an austerity program that began in 1972, the number of personnel decreased from 3,342 to 2,975 in 1973. This shift of personnel from hospital staff to corporate staff, which represented increased centralization of services, reflected the rapid growth of the system during these years. In 1968, the system consisted of Sun State Hospital and Eastham Hospital in a nearby city. By 1973, the system had grown to include eight hospitals in the metropolitan area

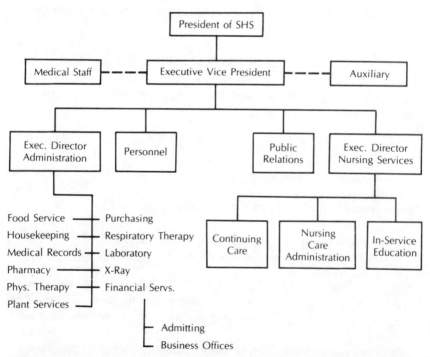

Figure 7.3. Presbyterian Hospital organization chart, August 1971.

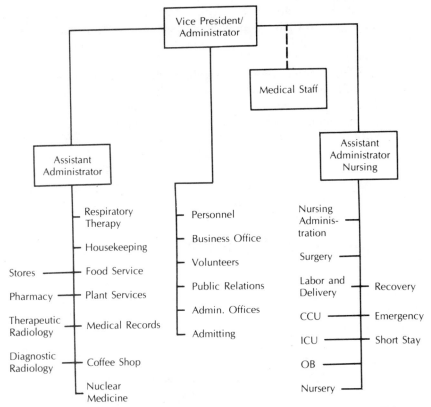

Figure 7.4. Presbyterian Hospital organization chart, May 1974.

and the north and northeastern parts of the state. Today, the system has six rather than eight inpatient facilities.

McLean himself admitted in 1971 that development had perhaps been too fast but that opportunities had presented themselves that might never again have been available.

Today, the system is run by McLean working closely with senior vice president David Williams. Williams handles internal problems, leaving McLean free to play a national role in health policy, and work on long-range planning for the system.

Summary

The SSHS has been characterized by the strong, aggressive management style of its chief executive officer. It operates in a geographic area that is highly competitive and is becoming more so.

The main incongruence within this system has been that of accelerated initial growth with a management poorly organized and unaware of the importance of legitimizing the system both to consumers and to other area providers.

While SSHS has had clearly articulated goals, it did not realize the potentially devastating effect of a powerful community group on these goals. Rather than developing gradually to allow relationships to be built among member institutions and within communities, SSHS expanded its corporate staff rapidly, with little attention to building confidence in SSHS and in multihospital systems as a whole. Although this incongruence led to a severe setback initially, it soon forced the management to reassess SSHS's goals and capabilities, creating in the long run a strengthened system.

METROPOLITAN MEDICAL CENTER

The Metropolitan Medical Center (MMC), founded in 1965, is geographically centralized, with all units located within ten miles of one another. There is little tradition of collaboration; in fact, there is a strong history of competition among the units that now make up the system. In addition, since the units are all full-facility units, there was even less incentive to work as a cohesive system than there might have been if the units had more need of each other's services.

Community groups as well as planning agencies have played a significant role in the development of this system, particularly in planning for expansion and in reorganizing facilities.

The other providers in the area have not presented a major stumbling block in the development of this system. The MMC is the principal provider of care in the region.

The vice president of finance handles capital financing. He supervises the comptroller responsible for general accounting, and a financial analysis group responsible for budgeting as well as cost-benefit analysis. The system also has a government reimbursement group that continuously reviews regulations in order to maximize reimbursement from third-party agencies. The diverse efforts the MMC has made to bolster its financial position are particularly interesting as a demonstration of the advantages to a system approach. It would be highly unusual for an independent community hospital to find the money needed to hire a reimbursement specialist or to undertake cost-benefit analysis. A system, on the other hand, can provide this kind of expertise.

The MMC, now the major medical and health care resource for its state, was formed by a merger of three voluntary, acute care general hospitals: the Bayview Hospital, the City Memorial Hospital, and the Doctors Hospital. The three hospitals are similar and traditionally have triplicated services and facilities.

All three faced the same problem troubling numerous other systems now developing: poor, urban populations need care more expensive and at a greater frequency than other populations. It is difficult to serve a poor, urban population, but even more difficult to desert it and move the institution away from the inner city into the suburbs. Responses to the problem have varied. Some systems have chosen to split services, providing certain services in one location and others at another. This has numerous logistic disadvantages, although it does avoid the problems of a "black–white" hospital. Another response is to maintain a "ghetto" hospital in the urban area, and subsidize it by a more profitable facility in the suburbs. This is also fraught with problems; it is difficult to attract qualified staff or willing consumers to an institution that is viewed as a "ghetto hospital." This in turn tends to lead to a deterioration in the care provided.

While the population served by the MMC has begun to move away from the inner city, the problem remains of what to do with the poor population still in urban ghettos. They resent being taken to the suburbs for care, and, of course, the suburban dwellers equally resent being brought into the downtown area for care. The problem has led to unrelieved tension among the three administrations, none of which can profitably exist on its own.

In 1965 a committee was formed to assess the feasibility of merger between three independent nonprofit hospitals. It had become evident to the boards that there was considerable triplication of programs and supplies, and that merger might be an attractive alternative. The chairman of the committee, George McGuire, was the person who conceptualized the merger and began to develop a strategy to implement it. It is interesting to note that as soon as the idea was realized, he left. Mr. Miller believes that it would have been impossible for the same person to stay on through the merger; previous research suggests strongly that the early direction and the later development can most easily be accomplished by different people.

When Mr. McGuire left, a university president was brought in who attempted to run the new medical center somewhat as he had run the university. After an interim period, Mr. Miller was recruited and entered the system shortly after management had become centralized. During this early period he felt that his principal job was to instill an increased sense of confidence in the new administration. After stabilizing the situation, Miller began to articulate a strategy and to implement it. This necessitated confrontation and negotiation, a task made more difficult by the previous leadership, which had led the medical staff to understand that the merger implied that all services would literally be under one roof. Miller's strategy, however, called for a redistribution of services so that care could be provided most effectively and efficiently, and he felt that these goals could best be met by separate facilities joined by adequate transportation. This led to planning a "two roof" institution, with one hospital in the city and one in the country, together serving the needs of both the urban population and the growing population in the southeast.[8]

Negotiation entailed a certain amount of secrecy, careful planning with members of the medical staffs and the board, and costly studies to prove the fiscal soundness of the "two roof" concept. The decision to split services was finally voted upon and approved by the medical staff and, according to Miller, "It was probably the first time the staff was together on anything." Miller accomplished this by working with coalitions of doctors and board members singly and in small groups, while at the same time sharing with them the cost estimates that were generated by his director of planning. A great deal of attention was given to the sequence of these meetings, as well as to who should attend, a factor which takes on importance in a small city such as Metropolitan's, where the board members in the chemical industry still have considerable power. These men, Miller says, were not the problem: "They're businessmen; if it looks like it is a logical plan, they're usually for it." The real problem was with those board members who had alliances to their own hospitals. But they were able to take a long-range view, a broad view, and to stop thinking provincially.

At the same time, the needs, and the perceived needs, of the neighborhood groups had to be addressed, and although Miller feels that the needs of the poor, black population are best met by dividing services, thereby ending a "black–white hospital," community leaders took considerably longer to be convinced. It is interesting to note that Miller did not sell this concept to community leaders himself, relying instead on other sympathetic community leaders to do it for him. While all of the CEOs interviewed noted that selling the system as the most efficient way to deliver care was a critical function today, Miller believes that the CEO is the least appropriate person to actually do the selling, since he inevitably is viewed as a biased party.

He views his role now less as a negotiator than as a consolidator, as someone whose responsibilities primarily include dealing with outside agencies and ensuring that the system can effectively react to these demands. While Miller monitors the impact of existing and potential environmental forces, his vice president for administration runs the day-to-day operations. The corporate staff is small and consists of a finance director, a public relations director, and a planning director. Unlike the other CEOs, Miller's travel is limited, perhaps because the system is still in an early evolutionary stage and his attention is needed on site more than at national meetings.

Summary

The collaborative climate in this city can best be described as antagonistic to the development of a multihospital system. Hospitals in the area have traditionally been protective of their own turf and hesitant to enter into collaborative agreements with outside institutions. In addition, pressure groups, particularly community groups, have played a major role in the development of MMC.

These environmental problems are not unique; emerging systems in other urban areas are often plagued by a similarly antagonistic environment. Yet the failure to adequately address these obstacles has often brought development to a standstill, particularly in an expanded suburban facility. To avoid this, significant efforts have been made since 1965 to strengthen the relationships among the three institutions in MMC; to encourage and facilitate bonds between trustees and medical staff; to strengthen the relationship with external regulatory agencies; and to secure financing for expansion. At the same time, little effort was made either to understand the potential power of community groups to affect the MMC's long-range planning, or to legitimize the system in their eyes. As a result, the system has reached a virtual standstill. Competent development in a variety of areas coupled with insufficient attention to legitimizing the system has created a degree of incongruence that has constrained further expansion.

SUMMARY

Each system operates in a unique environment, with certain characteristics of particular importance to the development of each system. In order to respond adequately to these external demands, the system must behave so as to:

achieve an appropriate alignment with the external environment, particularly to those five variables described in Chapter 6 that appear to be of particular importance: history of collaboration; existence and impact of local and regional pressure groups; geographical disper-

sion of units; competition with other providers; and scarcity of resources.

respond to environmental demands in a sequence that allows the
system to evolve. While a number of different tasks must be addressed, the sequence in which these tasks are addressed appears to
be a function of special demands of the environment in which the
system operates. One system, for example, may find it advantageous
to spend significant time establishing community alliances, while
another may find that developing a good relationship with community pressure groups must take second place to developing simple
and nonthreatening shared services with traditionally antagonistic
providers.

have a leader who is able to address these issues of alignment and
sequence. This person must exhibit different behavior and skills at
different times in the course of the system's development.

It seems clear, however, that each system diagnosed environmental
demands in a unique fashion and acted according to this assessment.
The Western Affiliated Hospital System, for example, operates in a
sophisticated and highly differentiated environment where a large
variety of health providers exists. It was clear that the system had to
develop an innovative product that would effectively distinguish it
from providers. This implicit strategy appears to have led to the establishment of a for-profit subsidiary.

Hillcrest Community Hospitals also operates in a sophisticated environment. Their innovation was the concept of the holding company,
one that proved useful locally as well as regionally to educate consumers about the system and consequently to legitimize it.

Sun State Health Service attempted a strategy for fast growth in
response to what it perceived as consumer demands. It did not, however, develop a product that was viewed as being distinctive, and it is
still trying to set itself apart from other area providers as well as from
other systems such as SJHHS who also operate in the area.

The Springvale Hospital System, on the other hand, did not have to
respond to preexisting environmental demands; when it was established it had the good fortune of being able to define its own role, and
by being responsive to constantly changing consumer needs, as well as
to the needs of other providers, it has been able to develop a preemptive
strategy.

The St. John's Hospitals and Homes Society appears to have had a
totally different strategy. Member units are located far from one another, tend to be small community institutions, and usually need the
efficiency and management expertise that SJHHS can provide by stan-

dardizing procedures. The system has made little effort to market its services; potential members seek out the system. The society can usually meet their primary needs—to remain financially viable so that they can continue to deliver care.

While Mid-Atlantic Regional Hospitals could have formulated and implemented a similar strategy of providing increased efficiency to its members, it chose to provide comprehensive health services to a population that was generally unable to pay for its own care. This strategy is an expensive one under the best of circumstances; in the depressed area served by MARH, a system that does not have a dependable source of revenue, it is unlikely to be successful.

Metropolitan Medical Center seems to be somewhat of an aberration; it has not been able to successfully address its central problem of efficiently providing care to a poor, urban population that is less than enthusiastic about receiving care in the suburbs. It has not developed a distinctive competence, and it is by no means clear that the establishment of the system has led to more efficient or effective delivery of care. Perhaps three autonomous hospitals with management agreements for certain services would have been more beneficial for consumers and staff. However, this system is still at an early developmental stage and, as a more mature system, it may well be able to deliver a service that is different from what consumers can now obtain.

NOTES

1. See Chapter 2 for a more thorough discussion of these traditional and continuing conflicts.
2. A particularly good example of a well-defined strategy is the following: Crown Cork and Seal aims to be a stripped-down and increasingly profitable manufacturer of specialty high-margin rigid containers for hard-to-hold applications (aerosol products and beer), and to maintain its position in bottling machinery and crowns. Its domestic growth will come from increasing the number of geographically decentralized small plants equipped and located to provide fast delivery at low transportation cost and to secure 20 percent to 40 percent of each local market. Customer service is led by a technically trained sales force alert to customer needs and by a technical "research" and manufacturing engineering organization solving current customer process and packing problems rather than doing basic research. Its current investment in innovation is kept small, but an aggressive marketing and a flexible manufacturing organization are alert to promote advances pioneered by major suppliers and competitors. Domestic operations are intended to be the stable base from which the company can expand internationally. The developing countries to which crown manufacture has already been introduced are expected to be the company's major growth opportunity in containers. Operations will be financed through retained earnings and full use of debt capacity and are expected to return twenty-five cents additional profit per share

per year. The organization will reward drive, energy, and accomplishment and accept rapid turnover in management ranks whenever results fall below expectations.

3. Reaching a workable compromise between allowing the independence of a unit and simultaneously being financially responsible for it remains an interesting problem.

4. As of January 1, 1978, Fisher became the CEO. Mr. Gardner now plays an active consulting job to the system and is spending most of his time on an institute to further the development of MHSs.

5. While an average number of E.R. visits for this size hospital cannot be given, 24,000 visits represents a particularly active emergency room.

6. In fact, nine out of ten requests for assistance are denied.

7. Coleman now travels about 70 to 80 percent of the time.

8. For example, between the 1960 and 1970 censuses, the home city lost 15,000 persons and its southeastern neighbor gained 10,000.

Chapter 8

Leadership Choices

INTRODUCTION

All of the systems studied appear to have effective leaders— executives who have, to varying degrees, understood the impact of the environment on their systems and who have formulated a complex set of responses.

While the methodological approach of this book has not been psychoanalytic or psychohistorical, the data suggest that a principal reason why these seven men have been effective in their roles has been their ability to:

diagnose the demands of the environment
perform certain activities in response to these demands
emphasize different skills at each developmental stage
   and during the transition periods between stages
maintain a workable equilibrium between personal needs and career
   demands

THE RELATIONSHIP BETWEEN
THE SYSTEM AND THE PERSON

The data suggest that as the system evolves, certain tasks must be executed. The nature of these tasks implies an emphasis on certain management skills rather than others. In an early stage, for example, when the purpose and goals of the system must be defined and shared, the chief executive officer must be an able arbitrator and negotiator. McLean said of this first stage that the necessary skills were those of bringing people together, of negotiating and promoting: "I personally negotiated every merger." During this stage political arbitration is another key skill. The CEO must know when to wait and do nothing, as Miller did at the Metropolitan Medical Center, when to forge ahead and begin to grapple with issues that are bound to be controversial, and when to concentrate on issues that are not likely to provoke argument in an effort to build confidence and trust. At a later stage, when for example critical decisions must be made concerning board membership and opening medical staff privileges, other skills must be emphasized, particularly those of confrontation and administration. Of the second stage McLean said, "We became a corporation during this period and I became a CEO rather than a hospital administrator." And finally, in the legitimizing stage, the CEO must step back from daily problems and ongoing events in order to effectively delegate. This stage emphasizes management, centralized services and program planning, with an emphasis on coordination among the different facilities. McLean says: "The important things to think about are what health care will look like in ten or twenty years." These varied roles demand a person who can, Janus-like, balance the interests of his own system and perhaps his own unit within that system, with the interests of other regional institutions.

While these tasks are required in order for the system to move forward, the person in the role of CEO may or may not be able to emphasize the needed skills. The CEO who is comfortable with a "hands on" approach in an early stage and finds that he can easily negotiate and confront, may find it significantly more difficult to achieve a "system" perspective during the legitimizing stage, which implies that he separate himself from daily activities, delegate much of his job, and maintain a low profile. Age as well as career stage may suggest that for a young person the activities typical of the earlier stages may be considerably more attractive. These factors notwithstanding, some managers are naturally "builders" who enjoy the earlier aspects of system evolution and gain little professional satisfaction from administrating an ongoing system, while other managers are more naturally "maintainers" who enjoy fine-tuning an existing system. Consequently, the fit between the necessary tasks implied by an evolving system and the psychological characteristics, age, and career stage of the chief executive officer must be congruent.

SITES

Hillcrest Community Hospitals is a particularly good example of these issues. At Hillcrest, while the tasks that Garrett has addressed have changed since the system was founded over twenty-five years ago, alterations have been responsive to both internal and external pressures, and Garrett's influence can be traced as a continuous thread throughout the development of the system. After being intimately involved with every aspect of operations, recent organizational changes suggest that Garrett is delegating authority and spending more time on the relationship of the system to its environment and to other systems than on daily operations. He sees himself playing a greater role in the financial arena and on long-term strategy while his two vice presidents increase their span of control. It is interesting to note that these major organizational changes are also accompanied by significant changes in Garrett's personal life, which have direct bearing on corporate strategy. Garrett has recently remarried; perhaps this remarriage, combined with his age (early fifties) and his personal goals, have made it easier to delegate more day-to-day operational decisions. He has chosen to shun constant breakfast meetings and views travel as a way to further his holding company concept, but as an activity that can often be done with his wife.

This is not to say that his style of management has significantly changed. He is a man who has carefully orchestrated his environment and he continues to do so. Critical decisions to be made at the quarterly board meetings are discussed at length in small groups before the meeting so that the larger meeting can be carefully controlled. This process appears to be universal in the systems studied, except in those systems where the board is not a force to contend with, such as the Springvale Hospital System where the board comprises seven people appointed by the legislature.

In short, Garrett is positive about the recent reorganization and feels that the changes will give him both the time he needs personally as well as the time to expand his system outside its present boundaries. To market Hillcrest effectively he feels he has to disassociate himself from Hillcrest Hospital ("I got to be known as Mr. Hillcrest") and become more of a regional and national leader so that he can have the credibility to significantly increase the number of institutions within the system and not be viewed as a partisan administrator who is only interested in "takeovers."

Garrett then has been able to emphasize different skills as the system evolved as well as to effectively combine his personal needs and abilities with those of his career.

Although Gardner, at Springvale Hospital System, is somewhat older than Garrett, there are also changes in his personal life which have made delegation increasingly easier. For the past few years he has felt exceedingly tired, and this fatigue proved to be not simply age-related but symptomatic of a heart condition, which was successfully operated on. Now he feels that he has additional strength and is even more interested in possible new directions for the system as well as for himself.

In order to work on these changes, Gardner has delegated "inside" responsibilities, yet still spends eight hours a day in meetings. He plays the role of environmental scanner and helps to diffuse accumulated information throughout the organization. The tasks that he has chosen to address have changed from the very specific, which revolved around adapting the mission of the system, to changing needs.

Jesse Lorrimer, president of the Western Affiliated Hospital Society, has developed a structure which has allowed him to gradually take a decreasing role as manager and become a full-time leader. In fact, he is, as of this writing, also playing a national leadership role as a member of the Board of Trustees of the American Hospital Association, a role which, as we have said, is connected to the third stage of development—the legitimizing stage—where the CEO finds it useful to "sell" the system to outsiders in order to establish confidence and trust regionally. His interests have moved away from the administrative sphere and into the area of long-term planning. He is concerned with capital financing, evolving regulatory policy, and the continuing development of not-for-profit subsidiaries. While Lorrimer continues to be concerned with the design of the system, the structure is such that strategic changes are likely to suggest gradual structural changes. Consequently he can take the time to address other issues.

Lorrimer expressed the same feelings as Garrett about the problems of making the transition between "inside" leader and "outside" leader. For him, the transition occurred when the corporate staff was formed and when he moved outside of the Golden State Hospital. He did this so that the staff would learn to not necessarily come to him. During the first few months he was aware of being extremely isolated; the move in fact represented the beginning of his job as CEO with a "system" perspective, rather than hospital administrator with a more parochial perspective.

Since the end of one stage and the beginning of another is seldom clearly marked by events, managing transition appears to be a particularly difficult task. Of the seven systems studied, four appear to be in a state of transition. Hillcrest is in the process of decentralizing operations as it begins to consider new methods of growth and expansion. The Metropolitan Medical Center is attempting to implement its "two roof" concept by building a large complex seven miles from the inner city and is being blocked by a civil rights power block. Mid-Atlantic Regional Hospitals must consider a drastic decrease in services if it cannot receive a government subsidy to make up some of the difference between revenue and expenses. At the same time, this system is also trying to decentralize its operations to give the communities more responsibility for their institutions. Springvale Hospital System has recently (January 1, 1978) gone through a major change; Craig Gardner is now assistant secretary to the board of trustees and is playing an active consultant role and becoming more involved nationally in multi-hospital systems, while Jack Fisher is the new general director. This does not imply that the other systems are static; by definition an MHS is dynamic and must remain responsive. These four, however, are in such an active stage of transition that the leaders are under special pressure.

The transition within the SHS is particularly interesting because Fisher's new position represents an attempt to deal with the issue of management succession, an issue the other systems have had some trouble addressing. Coleman is very much in total control at SJHHS, as is Lorrimer in WAHS, although Lorrimer makes ample use of his corporate managers who run the for-profit subsidiaries and is also serving in a national role.

The lack of attention to succession has, at Mid-Atlantic Regional Hospitals, for example, perhaps contributed to the system's problems. Each successive leader has had his own philosophy and his own interests, and appears to have actively pursued a new course while paying relatively little attention to the development of an ongoing and long-term financial strategy. Consequently, the present CEO, Dr. Dyer, is forced to play the role of crisis manager in order to address critical financial problems. In this system, as in other systems that are in transition, the skills needed are those of mediation and negotiation; regardless of the natural proclivity of the CEO to be an innovator rather than an implementor, transition usually demands a hands-on manager.

In all of these systems, the CEO must generate and use power. In *The Executive Role Constellation*,[1] where three executives at a mental hospital are studied, the authors believe that, in order to generate and use the necessary power, executives become involved in a network of interpersonal transactions in striving to realize organizational objectives. In order to generate power, the executive commits himself to a series of reciprocal transactions related to organizational objectives. Influence is generated as a result of these transactions, which allows the executive to affect the course of events within the organization as well as its future. This is not an immediate process; it is time consuming and its success is difficult to assess until a situation occurs that tests the level of power and the executive's ability to utilize it. In other words, both organizational and personal factors are involved in an executive's generation and use of power, and the process of learning takes place over the course of the executive's career in a series of what Hodgson, et al. call "person–position resolutions." Given the number of power bases that the CEO of an MHS must take into account, this concept of reciprocal relationships seems to be a particularly appropriate way to describe what the CEO does within such a system. In addition, these system leaders play a broader role in relating to state and national organizations. Finally, they relate to other systems and other facilities either by free or purchased consulting services.

SUMMARY

The issue of leadership is one that interests a great many system managers, perhaps because it is unclear what kind of leader would most effectively manage an emerging MHS in contrast to one at a more mature stage of development. The data gathered in the course of this study suggest that personal abilities, professional background, and the specific characteristics of a particular system are all critical variables that must be addressed. While consistency of leadership is advisable, if the leader cannot or will not adapt his behavior to changing demands, a change in leadership appears preferable to a rigidity of behavior. While there appear to be certain skills required at different stages of development, these skills must be congruent with the needs and ability of the CEO as well as with the needs of the system.

NOTE

1. Hodgson, Levinson, and Zaleznick, *Executive Role Constellation.*

Chapter 9

Conclusions

INTRODUCTION

A variety of collaborative arrangements among hospitals have emerged during the past few decades as financial and regulatory pressures have made it increasingly difficult for many hospitals to operate independently. Collaborations today take many innovative forms, which may represent an attempt by health care providers to respond to pressure in a way that maximizes their existing strengths and minimizes loss of autonomy.

This book has concentrated on formal collaborative arrangements that are managed by a chief executive officer and has explored the development of seven major multihospital systems.

In Chapter 3, four questions were proposed:

1. Is there a relationship between the age of the system and its organizational effectiveness?
2. Are there environmental variables relevant to all MHSS?
3. Are system responses related to environmental demands and do they change over time?
4. What is the relationship between the chief executive officer and the development of each system?

These questions suggested certain relevant areas in the literature, some of which appeared useful in analyzing the data obtained at the seven sites. The factors that have been explored in some depth as "environmental factors" and "system responses" suggest four hypotheses, one relating to each of the research questions that were originally posed. In this chapter, we will first discuss these four hypotheses and then propose an exploratory model which relates them to one another. Figure 9.1 describes graphically the relationship between the research questions and the literature review.

THE HYPOTHESES

The data collected at the seven sites suggest four hypotheses:

1. The age of a system is likely to have a strong impact on its ability to diagnose environmental demands and develop in a way that appropriately addresses these demands.
2. Environmental demands can be characterized in such a way that they are relevant to all multihospital systems.
3. Each system responds to environmental demands in a way that is congruent with the peculiar nature of these demands and the relative salience of each.
4. The skills of the CEO and the tasks he addresses are a function of the demands on the system and change over time.

Hypothesis #1: The Age of a System Is Likely to Have a Strong Impact on Its Ability to Diagnose Environmental Demands and to Develop in a Way That Appropriately Addresses These Demands

While most of the research on multihospital systems has been descriptive, a number of variables have been postulated to explain the growth of a system in a particular geographic area where a number of providers continue to operate independently.

In the major work on multihospital systems done by the American Hospital Association in 1974, the director of the study, James Cooney, hypothesizes that the age of the system can perhaps explain why one system seems to be relatively free of organizational problems while another continues to be troubled. He concludes that the age of the system is critical; that the internal trauma of organizational change brought on by the formation of a multihospital system is lessened by age.

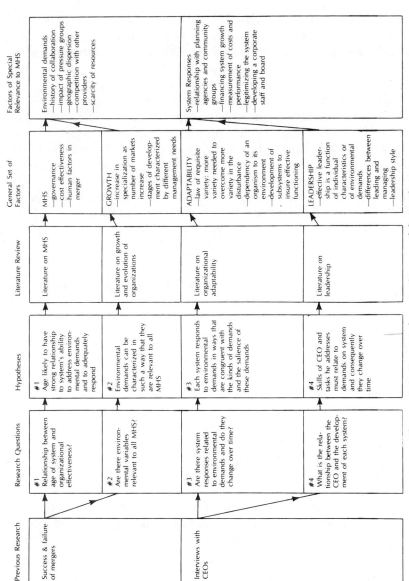

Figure 9.1. Research questions and hypotheses.

145

I have addressed the question of age during the course of this book. The data suggest that there does appear to be a strong relationship between the age of the system and its ability to effectively diagnose and adapt to its environment, although one cannot necessarily predict the effectiveness of the system from its chronological age. One system can spend many years performing a particular activity, such as strengthening its relationships with regulatory agencies, while another can go on quickly to other issues, such as increasing the scope of its services in order to broaden its revenue base. Yet a sequence of activities does appear to exist, and data suggest that the nature of these activities changes as the system evolves. This evolution can be described in terms of broad stages, a concept that has been useful in the private sector to compare companies within the same industry. Data suggest three stages of development for an MHS:

1. The building or establishment stage, characterized by issues of joining, membership, governance, and financial viability. There is usually a principal agent or "prime mover" quite visible during this early stage, who tends to be the chief executive officer of an institution but can be an external force, such as a state legislature.
2. The solidifying stage, characterized by attention to the issues of the building stage. However, during this stage the emphasis is on internal work, especially on the part of the CEO, rather than external work. While attention must constantly be paid to the relationship of the system's component parts to its environment, the solidifying stage involves developing and training the corporate staff, addressing issues of interdependence and communication among the units, and learning from earlier mistakes.
3. The legitimizing stage, characterized by an emphasis on building a strong reputation and selling system capabilities to potential system members. During this stage the mature system begins to feel comfortable with its internal mechanisms and may play a pivotal role both regionally and nationally in the formulation of health care policies.

Unfortunately, there are no clear signals by which a system knows that it is ready to go from one stage to another; entering the legitimizing stage, for example, when internal mechanisms are not yet solidified, can prove to be problematic. An approximation of the seven systems along the spectrum of developmental stages and their chronological age can be found in Figure 9.2.

Since placement along this spectrum is clearly a subjective judgment, some justification seems warranted. The Metropolitan Medical

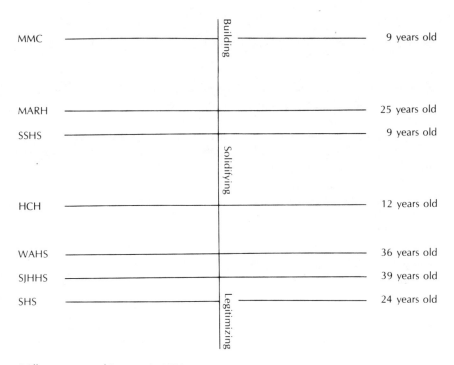

^a All ages are as of January 1, 1974.

MMC: Metropolitan Medical Center
MARH: Mid-Atlantic Regional Hospitals
SSHS: Sun State Health Service
HCH: Hillcrest Community Hospitals
WAHS: Western Affiliated Hospital Society
SJHHS: St. John's Hospitals and Homes Society
SHS: Springvale Hospital System

Figure 9.2. Developmental stages.

Center (MMC) is clearly in a building phase. Although the system is nine years old,[1] the time has largely been spent on establishing relationships among critical institutions so that collaboration would eventually flow more smoothly. The results of earlier research that explored the early development of collaborative systems that were noncorporate in structure is relevant here.[2] It was found that in the early stages of collaboration, meetings were needed to insure that the different parties would begin to communicate. The substance of these meetings was almost inconsequential; the important issue was that critical players who had traditionally said little to one another were now interacting. These early meetings often addressed topics that at first glance seemed superficial,[3] such as the development of the forms that were to be used for a particular kind of diagnosis. But these meetings in themselves, regardless of the content, proved to be a critical first step. Thus for the MMC early collaboration may eventually prove instrumental to the development of the system. In fact, the system has already made considerable progress. Three traditionally separate hospitals came together, and perhaps some of the institutional energies that had historically been spent on competition are now being spent on activities that will benefit broad segments of the community, such as building satellite neighborhood outreach facilities tied together by a transportation system. At the time of this writing, however, further movement for this system has been momentarily stopped as a result of unsolved and long-standing disputes between the system proponents who wish to build a new facility outside the inner city, and civil rights activists who wish to keep full service facilities in the urban area. It is difficult to say how this problem might have been avoided. Clearly, it did not help to have a transition in leadership at a critical point. Data also suggest that an effective job of boundary scanning was not done; the potential impact of civil rights activists appears to have been underestimated.

Mid-Atlantic Regional Hospitals (MARH) is next on the spectrum. This system has consistently been idealistic in its objectives and somewhat unrealistic in its lack of long-term financial strategy. Again, the system has been hampered by changes in leadership at various critical developmental points. These changes, coupled with a lack of attention to the development of a dependable revenue base, has severely restricted the forward movement of the system. In an effort to adapt to changing environmental conditions, MARH has tried to decentralize operations to encourage community support, but inattention to the critical task of becoming financially solvent has all but stopped this system, and has certainly affected the number of available services.

In fact, MARH can be considered the one "deviant" in this relationship between age and developmental stages. Rather than moving from the building stage to solidifying and then to legitimizing, MARH has been hindered in its development by two principal factors: its close relationship to UMW, which curtails its revenue at unexpected points, creating a high level of uncertainty unique to this system, and the large number of indigent patients, which makes it difficult for MARH to implement its strategy of a comprehensive health and illness system.

Sun State Health Service, the next on the spectrum, appears to be in a solidifying stage. Rapid early growth not coupled with the establishment of an efficient structure to effectively control the growth, as well as a lack of attention in the early years to building strong community support, led to serious obstacles for this system. However, these obstacles, specifically the corporation controversy, led to valuable reorganization that has resulted in a decrease in the size of the corporate staff, a greater rapport with the community, and a growth strategy that addresses the needs of the region and the abilities of the corporate staff. The leadership within this system has been consistent and competent; McLean clearly commands respect from his staff as well as from regional and national leaders. It could be argued that, had it not been for this consistency, the problems experienced by this system might have proven far more serious.

Hillcrest Community Hospitals (HCH) has passed through a solidifying stage during which critical changes were made in the structure. Garrett now shares his leadership role and has begun to delegate more effectively while taking on the role of long-range planner. The system, which now consists of three owned institutions as well as extensive management contracts, is at the stage where attention must be paid to its long-term development, including growth, financing, and the role of its board. At the same time, a competent internal management has been developed, freeing Garrett's time.

Western Affiliated Hospital Society (WAHS), St. John's Hospitals and Homes Society (SJHHS), and Springvale Hospital System (SHS) are all in a mature stage of development. What immediately differentiates SHS from the other two is that attention has been paid to management succession; Gardner has been succeeded by Fisher. This issue of succession is a complicated one. The leader of an MHS must have a broad perspective; there is considerable difference between an institutional leader and a system leader. It is difficult to have both of these perspectives; it is even more difficult to train a subordinate so that he or she develops a "system" perspective while at the same time learns to manage or to supervise the management of complex operations. For this reason, having two people at the helm, one playing an internal leadership role and the other playing an external and a planning role, may be the best solution. This is what SHS has been doing; now the situation has been altered in that Gardner is moving away from the immediate concerns of the system. It is unclear whether Fisher will play the same external role, deciding what new areas the system should explore and keeping a close watch on environmental demands that could affect the system.

While WAHS has not made such a clear distinction between the internal and external leaders, Lorrimer extensively uses the services of his corporate managers who operate the for-profit subsidiaries. He appears to have consciously and effectively made the transition from institutional leader to system leader and is now spending a significant amount of his time in the legitimizing function, both regionally and nationally. Like SSHS, and of course all the systems to varying degrees, WAHS has made mistakes; expansion was not always as well planned as it might have been. But again like SSHS, it has apparently reached an equilibrium between level of growth and the necessary corporate structure.

The SJHHS is clearly a mature system, one that has been able to break many decisions down into their programmable component parts so that ninety units can be run by a small corporate staff. The system has also reached a unique level of sophistication in that it operates in sixty-five different communities and manages to remain responsive to their varied environmental demands. The question of management succession, however, has not been addressed, and since Clarence Coleman appears to operate the system almost singlehandedly, it remains to be seen what will happen when he retires.[4]

Hypotheses #2 and #3: Each System Responds to Environmental Demands in a Way That Is Congruent with the Peculiar Nature of These Demands and the Relative Importance of Each

It appears, then, that for the system to move forward, each stage implies certain activities that are a function of specific external demands. Figure 9.3 depicts this relationship: while all activities and all skills are of course necessary in every stage, the question is one of emphasis.

The First Stage: Building the System. While each stage is characterized by many of the same activities, certain activities are emphasized as the system develops. During the first stage, for example, special attention must be given to the following activities:

diagnosing the environment
clarifying the financial philosophy
defining the appropriate decision process
dealing with conflict resolution
organizing the corporate staff
integrating the member units

During the first stage the system must understand what environmental factors are of particular importance. If, for example, there are a number of other providers in the area, then broadening services that imply a change in referral patterns is likely to cause problems. If

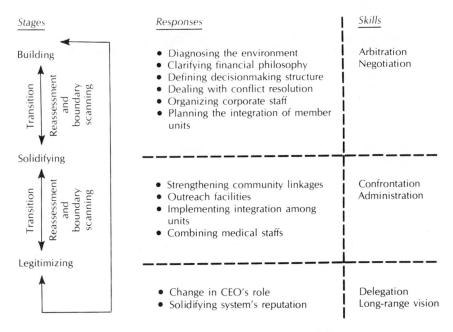

Figure 9.3. Stages, responses, and skills.

consumer expectations in the area are such that closing an unprofitable unit will be met with significant resistance, then it might be more advisable to live with this unprofitability and attempt the change at a later point when relationships are more firmly established. Because each environment is so different, what might be acceptable behavior for a health provider in one area may be unacceptable in another. HCH, for example, transported patients from one unit to another in order to avoid duplication of facilities. MMC would meet considerable resistance doing the same thing. In a similar vein, malpractice appears to be a much more important issue in the urban northeast than it is in the rural midwest.

Other tasks also need to be addressed during the initial developmental phase. It is useful for the system to articulate its overall financial philosophy. Is each unit to be financially self-sufficient, or is one purpose of the system to support "losing" units? A number of points are of course possible along this continuum; like other issues which the CEO must address, it is unfortunately not black or white. HCH believed in subsidizing the operations of Hillcrest–Willowdale while the unit came "on-line." After that point it was to be self-sufficient. MMC was to subsidize the operations of the urban unit on a long-term basis while operating a large suburban complex.

Another task during this period is that of defining an appropriate decisionmaking process. If decisions are to be made by voting, then how can the CEO encourage the "no-sayers" to be supportive when they voted against an action? If decisions are to be reached by consensus, and multiple boards exist, then the process is likely to be so cumbersome that forward movement will effectively be stopped. Consensus also suggests frequent contact among the principal actors so that the CEO can gauge when the group has reached consensus.[5]

Conflict resolution must also be addressed, since conflicts are bound to occur. If a certain unit consistently plays a "smoothing" role and avoids confrontation but does not feel accountable for its actions, the CEO must address this problem.

A decision must also be made internally about the size and the training of the corporate staff. Rather than immediately addressing this task, data suggest that existing staff should take on corporate functions until the purposes of the system are well established. The risk of building an extensive corporate staff at the wrong time is high; the community may feel that since a corporate staff exists to do the necessary work, little commitment is demanded of them. It would seem that a small staff is best, working closely with the CEO. A common pattern is that of Mr. Miller at MMC, who has a director of planning and a director of finance as well as a vice president for medical affairs. He works closely with Harold Davis, a man four or five years his junior who was with the system before 1971 when Mr. Miller became the CEO. In a similar vein, Craig Gardner has worked closely with Jack Fisher, who has been entirely in charge of operational matters and who is, in fact, his successor. Donald Dyer at MARH has decreased his corporate staff significantly since he took over the system and now has two vice presidents rather than five, but also relies on a small corporate staff.

While the obvious agenda for each member institution (such as achieving financial solvency), is usually evident in this first stage, one of the critical early responses on the part of the CEO and his staff is to understand the motives that each unit has for becoming part of the system and what it hopes to gain from the relationship. While each unit must want to join, it must be remembered that if it could receive the perceived benefits on its own, it would remain autonomous. This suggests a conflict that is difficult to avoid between the needs of the units and those of the system. While this conflict cannot be avoided, its potential risks can be reduced. Norms must be established regarding relative strength and equality among the units. For example, if the financially weak facilities are continually referred to as the "little" hospitals, if the competence of each institution is not taken into account, if the smaller institutions are clearly viewed as unequal by having fewer votes, problems are bound to develop. In other words, the relationship among member units, each of whom joined the system for different reasons, must be addressed.

The Second Stage: Solidifying the System. During the second stage, certain activities must be emphasized:

strengthening community linkages
addressing the need for outreach facilities
implementing the integration of the units
combining medical staffs

The second stage is characterized by solidifying previously made arrangements. Community linkages must be strengthened either by means of using advisory boards, as SHS did, or by using community councils or functional boards. Lorrimer of WAHS feels that, although a single board structure is clearly easier to handle, the multiple and interlocking board structure he uses is more effective in establishing strong roots in each community and in strengthening the power of the individual administrators who report to their own boards as well as to him. During this stage, the need for outreach or intake facilities should be addressed. The reasons for this are complex: as a system becomes viewed as having power, it is usually viewed as being solvent regardless of its actual financial condition. This in turn leads to community expectations that the system should be able to do "more" for the community. Teaching hospitals face the same problem. In many cities, among them Chicago and Boston, well-known teaching hospitals are often viewed as not being responsive to the communities in which they are located. High consumer expectations lead to the establishment of outreach facilities such as neighborhood health centers or clinics, as well as extensive ambulatory care facilities; all these represent serious demands on the institution.

MHSs face a similar problem. There is often pressure on a system to take care of the indigent and to continue the operation of non-revenue-producing services; it becomes difficult to sort out what should be done to improve accessibility of care while simultaneously remaining efficient. In some systems, such as the MARH, this involvement with outreach facilities was clearly proactive and did not come about as a result of community pressure. Efforts have been made all along within this system to provide home care and extended care, and in effect to provide in situ care to a population that did not demand it.

Another task during this stabilization stage is to define and implement the necessary integration among the units. Geography plays a critical part in this decision. For the SJHHS, the units are so far apart that integration is not an issue. The traditional effort within this system has been to centralize as many decisions as possible; this effort appears to have been appropriate. Effective integration is not only difficult to establish in a broad geographical area, but is seldom viewed as being necessary by the units themselves. However, in an area where the units are close to one another, such as MMC, integration becomes a critical and a difficult issue. It becomes imperative to set up mechanisms to facilitate interaction among the principal actors in order that the participants can begin to have a systems perspective and a sense of shared values. Task forces and other committees are not useful in themselves unless they are structured in such a way that involvement by all relevant parties actually takes place and that the results of these meetings affect all institutions. The systems studied tended to put little emphasis on the way in which the units related to one another. Perhaps attention to such coordination is more likely to come at a later stage of development, but these seven systems placed considerably more emphasis on developing the singular competence of each facility rather than on the interrelationships among the units. Even when communication is emphasized, the concern is to maximize the flow of information from the units to the headquarters (Figure 9.4a) and back, rather than among the units (Figure 9.4b).

Perhaps the mechanism the SSHS uses is typical. A corporate officer's meeting is held every two to three weeks. This meeting tends to be rather informal. Participants, including Mr. McLean and the corporate vice presidents as well as the hospital administrators, are encouraged to "brainstorm." Once each month a more formal meeting is held. In addition to the people who attend the corporate officers' meeting, this meeting of the executive council includes the risk man-

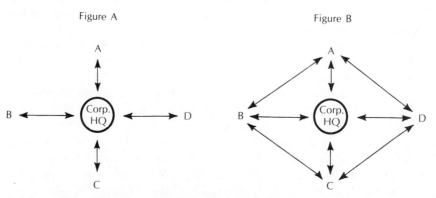

Figure A   Figure B

Figure 9.4. Differential information flow.

ager and Janet Borel, assistant to Mr. McLean. These two meetings tend to address all issues that could affect the component parts of the system.

An additional issue during this stabilization stage is that of combining medical staff. This possibility is of course contingent on geography; if the units are far from one another, open staff privileges are not realistic. But the issue is a complicated one for other reasons as well. If the medical staff has "open" privileges, the weaker institutions often fear that they will lose patients to those institutions that may have more "state of the art" facilities. Once feelings arise concerning a possible loss of patients, problems are likely in other areas. The question needs to be addressed, but it appears most useful to do so when other relationships have been well established.

The Third Stage: Legitimizing the System. During this stage the following activities need to be emphasized:

change in the CEO's role
solidifying the system's reputation

In the third stage it becomes particularly important for the CEO to separate himself from the crisis management approach that is often appropriate during the first two phases and to begin developing an internal leader while he takes more of a consultant–advisor–listener stance. This change does not imply that he separates himself from operations. In fact, it may mean that he attends just as many meetings but finds ways to use his time more effectively so that he can remain involved while not playing a pivotal role in every day-to-day event. Craig Gardner, at the SHS, for example, has a simple technique:

> When we meet, everyone has their own items on the agenda, but then after the meeting I ask them to send me a memorandum based on the notes they took at the meeting, which I then turn over to my secretary, who puts it into what's called a 'tracking sheet.' These sheets are simply items that are discussed and which still need to be resolved or which need additional work, and the tracking sheet of each person is the basis on which I follow through with the material that we covered in our conference—what we decided had to be done, who was to do it, and under what conditions.

Gardner feels that this is particularly useful in that it gives him a memo that comes from each person "so that I have the opportunity to find out if in fact they heard the same thing I heard, and if in fact it was the same thing." If the system is in transition this task of effectively organizing one's time becomes difficult, if not impossible, to accomplish. Dr. Dyer and Mr. Miller, at MARH and MMC, do not have the luxury of sitting back and taking a good look at past activities while at the same time planning future ones; the needs of their systems are such that planning must take a subordinate role to the resolution of immediate problems.

During this stage, the system must solidify its reputation regionally and nationally. This is not merely important for public relations reasons. It is also important for fundraising reasons and to gradually build allegiance to the system as a whole rather than to the individual units. It is difficult, for example, for the average consumer to understand the reasons for closing a unit. The inconvenience becomes a critical factor when hospital visits have to be made. Although the inconvenience will continue to exist, if the community has been educated to have confidence in the management of the system, the inconvenience associated with a decision is likely to decrease in importance compared to the perceptions about the quality of care or the extent of available services.

Care must also be taken not to "oversell" the consumer by letting him believe that collaboration necessarily implies cost savings. Economic studies suggest that if and when savings do occur, it takes years to happen. Cost containment rather than reduction is a more realistic possibility, but even this is difficult to assess. The system should be legitimized on grounds that can be defended by providers and understood by consumers, such as reduced duplication, more modern technology, physician cooperation, and the availability of increased funding. It is interesting to note that while some of the CEOs interviewed, such as Lorrimer, believed that legitimizing the system was one of their principal roles, others, particularly Miller, felt that this function can best be performed by other people who are respected within the community, but are not viewed as "system spokespeople." On a national level, legitimization is equally important; if the development of MHSs does lead to cost containment, reduced duplication of services, and more rational delivery of care, then the development of a national health policy that encourages such collaboration will only come about if the systems become well known. Again, the ability of the CEO to absent himself is a function of how well the previous tasks have been addressed. Most important perhaps in this stage is evaluation of what has been done, and assessment of new roles that the system might play. This involves self-study as well as an understanding of community and regional needs. It sometimes leads to a change of direction such as an emphasis on the problems of the geriatric population within the MHS, to a decrease in facilities such as closing a clinic that does not serve a large enough population, or to a reorganization of top management such as HCH did.

Hypothesis #4: Skills of CEO and the Tasks He Addresses Must Relate to External Demands and Change over Time

While all stages appear to require those characteristics usually associated with competent leadership, such as the ability to motivate subordinates and plan future activities, each stage appears to require an emphasis on certain skills.

The First Stage: Building the System. The CEO must emphasize his abilities to arbitrate and negotiate in the early stages when decisions are being made about membership and overall purpose and goals. This early role of strategist and politician is a difficult one; it is not a role that can be learned quickly. Speed can even be detrimental, for it often precludes the development of trust among existing and potential members. Timing is a critical ingredient during this early phase. If participants are rushed into making decisions, research suggests that they will not feel accountable for them, and may in fact stop further negotiations. If, on the other hand, decisions are not made, it is difficult to move from one stage to another.

The Second Stage: Solidifying the System. During the solidification stage, skills of confrontation are particularly important. At this point, critical parties are likely to have made a commitment to the system as a whole. Decisions will have been made about such issues as board representation, or the relationship between the number of votes and the division of assets. It is appropriate for the CEO to confront those units that are not conforming to previously made decisions. He must also be an administrator during this phase. While this skill, like the others, is always necessary, it becomes important to stabilize the relationships made earlier and to work with the existing mechanisms—in effect, to maintain the status quo until further refinements prove to be necessary. Yet, as the system grows, refinements are often required. The coordination that worked effectively among five units may not work for ten units, or even for seven units.

The Third Stage: Legitimizing the System. The third stage is marked by a need for the ability to delegate and provide "vision." As the CEO pulls away from daily crises, he must attempt to develop a long-range perspective and an innovative view of what the system might do. In order to do this, he must have learned to delegate in a way that is comfortable both to him and to his managers. Delegation does not mean desertion; in an MHS it is particularly important for the CEO to remain in contact with daily decisions while setting aside time for planning and reflection. This skill is particularly difficult to develop because the men who manage these systems are hospital administrators; they are skilled in, and appear to enjoy, crisis management. It is often counterintuitive for them to separate themselves from daily activities and to become reflective, yet maintaining the status quo during this third stage is usually inappropriate. Without innovation, adaptation is unlikely to occur. If enlarging the system becomes an issue at this point, it becomes particularly important to have regional as well as national acceptance and to refine operations so that financial viability is ensured. Provisions should be made for new activities to be pinpointed, evaluated, and possibly added. Often this environmental scanning appears to go hand in hand with the legitimizing function: as the CEO travels—often a necessary activity during this stage—he comes into contact with new ideas which can then be applied to his own system.

CHARACTERISTICS AND USE
OF THE MODEL

It seems clear then that the four proposed hypotheses help to explain the development of MHSs. Age clearly has an effect on the ability of a system to decide what environmental factors have to be attended to and which ones can wait. This diagnostic skill is critical so that the system can develop appropriate responses.

Although each system operates in a unique environment, there do appear to be common factors that must be attended to. The activities that each system chooses in order to respond to those factors that are of particular significance make up the system's strategy. These activities change over time, just as the strength and importance of the external demands change over time. In a similar vein, the role the CEO plays must change in order to insure an appropriate level of congruence between external demands and system responses. (See Figure 9.4 on page 154.)

It appears, then, that a useful model that can describe the development of the MHS and can predict where problems are likely to occur in the evolution of a system must include:

information concerning aspects of the environment relevant to the development of a hospital system

responses initiated by the system's management to address environmental demands

a range of skills that the CEO must have or develop in order to address changing environmental needs and system responses

In order for such a model to explain the development of a particular system rather than to simply describe the development of such systems in general, a number of linkages or connections need to be made among the component parts of the model: the environment, the range of available responses, and the need for certain skills rather than others. Each system must achieve a level of congruence among component parts of the model. It is this congruence which makes the different parts of the model work together as a unified whole.

If, for example, the system is in the building stage in an environment where:

there is little history of collaboration
considerable competition among providers
the units the system comprises are close together, suggesting a high need for integration

and the chief executive officer is at a point in his life where he wants more time to himself, fewer breakfast meetings, and in general, an increased separation between his personal and professional life, then problems are likely to ensue. This lack of congruence between the needs of the CEO and the stage of development that calls for a high investment of time in order to successfully arbitrate among providers and negotiate decisions that will allow the system to evolve into the later stages, means that the needs of the system are unlikely to be sufficiently addressed.

In a similar vein, a young CEO who is anxious to further his career and is willing to spend the necessary time attending to the needs of the developing system may find it difficult to emphasize the needs of the system as a whole rather than the needs of the corporate headquarters. In this early stage, the CEO often finds it important to keep a relatively low profile and develop the identity of member units, a task which is difficult for the younger, ambitious administrator who chafes at maintaining a low profile either institutionally or personally.[6]

In addition, the trait of being a "builder," someone who enjoys putting a system together, or a "maintainer," someone who enjoys taking over an established system at a later time, seldom appear in the same person. Yet a "builder" often finds it difficult to delegate, just as a "maintainer" finds it difficult to arbitrate among parties with conflicting goals. This problem suggests that unless the CEO in question can increase the scope of his interests and skills as the system develops, perhaps a different person should manage the system at a later stage of development.

The matrix of possible linkages between environment characteristics, available system responses, and necessary skills is too broad for a specific example of each situation. However, a comparison of two hypothetical systems, A and B, might be useful to illustrate the use of this exploratory model. System A could operate in an environment that has:

a strong history of collaboration
minimal competition among providers, perhaps because their needs
   are interdependent
broad geographical dispersion and low impact of pressure groups

This would suggest the need for a person who was a capable administrator and able to delegate. If, however, one of these variables were to change—let us say that pressure groups had recently become much more powerful in the area as a result of racial conflict that had begun to have a "spillover" effect on the delivery of health care—then the CEO would have to be a capable arbitrator as well as an administrator. This new combination of skills might suggest a different person for System B.

In order to look at the necessary congruence between the system's environment and the appropriate range of responses, it would be useful to use the same example. The environment of System A would suggest far more attention to making the purpose and goals clear than to the decisionmaking apparatus: if the units are unlikely to be working closely together on a daily basis because of their location, and if there is little history of competition among providers, then as long as members were clear as to how they were to relate to the corporate headquarters and as to what membership in the system was likely to do for them, then constantly scanning the environment or developing a decisionmaking mechanism based on consensus rather than a majority vote is less important. In the case of System B, however, where the one altered variable in the environment is an increased impact of community groups, the situation would be considerably different. Now, the critical issue might be to decide on appropriate levels of indigent care[7] in order to reduce racial tension and to incorporate community representatives into the decisionmaking structure.

In this example the two systems are similar except for a change in one variable. Yet responses must be quite different in order to achieve an appropriate level of congruence between the demands of the environment, the responses of the system, and the skills of the CEO, thus illustrating the complexity of system development. Yet it also illustrates the applicability of this exploratory model: if an appropriate analysis is made of the relevant environmental variables and enough is known about the existing and potential skills of the CEO, then a necessary level of congruence can be achieved among component parts of the model. An interested researcher or administrator can use the model to devise a workable set of activities given "X" environment that may have to be adjusted as one or more variables in "X" environment changes.

The implications of such a model for administrators and academicians as well as for the health system as a whole will be explored more fully in the final chapter.

NOTES

1. Age as of January 1, 1974.
2. The development of a cancer cooperative in Western Massachusetts, organized in order to make high quality cancer treatment available to a larger population at an earlier point in the disease process, by means of a collaboration among providers.
3. It is interesting to note that a common topic of early meetings among potential collaborators is often a shared laundry, perhaps because it is usually easy to agree on the issue and consequently, the parties can begin to talk to one another with a minimum amount of antagonism.
4. Retirement could, in this case, have numerous meanings. He might, for example, decide that he no longer wishes to spend 70 to 80 percent of his time travelling, and this change would necessitate a significant alteration in the kind of work that he delegates and in the necessary competence of his corporate staff. It could also mean total separation from the system. In either case, it is not clear how adaptable the system would be to such a change.
5. One hospital merger situation, involving several institutions, will serve as an example. According to the terms of the merger, each hospital's board of trustees had to ratify each decision before it could be implemented. The "speed" of decisionmaking was thus so slow that by the time any consensus was achieved, factors in the environment had changed and the decision was out of date. Over the course of a decade, several successive leaders tried, without success, to bring the new institutional relationship to fruition. Finally, in 1974, a new administrator was chosen. He saw what was wrong and designed a new decisionmaking system. By using a smaller group of decisionmakers and limiting the type of decisions that needed general approval, he circumvented the cumbersome multiboard machinery and was able to respond quickly to environmental issues. Within a year after he had assumed leadership, the merger had come to life.
6. An interesting example comes to mind: I held a number of interviews with leaders of noncorporate systems. One of these men runs a large consortium on the east coast. When I asked if he could be interviewed and if that interview could perhaps be used for a new health care journal, he declined, saying that he would be willing to speak about his experiences as CEO of the consortium in private, for research purposes. However, he felt that if he were to be interviewed in a nationally read journal as "Mr. Consortium," it would significantly affect the development of the system because he had expended considerable energy diminishing his seeming importance and maximizing the apparent importance of the executives within member institutions.
7. Beyond regulated levels that are imposed on the organization.

Chapter 10

Implications

INTRODUCTION

A significant change in the character of an industry tends to have broad implications for those people within the industry who are likely to be affected by the changes, for consumers who purchase the end products, and for researchers who try to learn from the changes.

I have examined such a change by studying the development of seven multihospital systems. I will discuss implications from the vantage point of the following:

administrators whose institutions are considering joining a system
administrators whose institutions are already part of a system
researchers who study organizational development
the health system as a whole

IMPLICATIONS FOR HOSPITAL ADMINISTRATORS

During the past decade, the administrator of an average-sized institution has had to significantly increase the numbers and kinds of people with whom he interacts. While these contacts have traditionally been limited to trustees, community agencies, and consumer groups, today regulatory groups and planning agencies demand a great deal of his time.

Today, in fact, the bulk of the administrator's attention is occupied by issues that are external in nature, whereas a few years ago these issues were of relatively minor importance.[1] Increased collaboration is one such issue. Yet few administrators are aware of the many implications of a multihospital system:

• Administrators can use an awareness of the different stages to adapt their own behavior and that of their subordinates to the demands of each stage. During the earlier stages, effective internal management implies an ability to negotiate numerous contracts and informal relationships. The nature of these relationships should take environmental demands into account. For example, a CEO whose system has been characterized by consistent involvement of community groups and by a limited history of collaboration must spend more time nurturing community relationships, including consumer education, than a CEO whose system faces other environmental pressures.

As the system evolves it usually becomes clear that the CEO can no longer effectively diagnose changing environmental demands, hire and train a corporate staff, attend all relevant meetings, and make operational decisions. At this point, an internal leader coupled with an external leader appears to work most effectively. Consequently, the stage of the system suggests those skills that a manager should have, and his level of involvement with internal as opposed to external affairs. These in turn suggest that the age of the CEO might be a critical factor. While there are of course exceptions, the changing demands of the position imply that a young person who is trying to establish himself in the field may find that keeping a low profile is difficult, while an older person may find this to be an easier task.

This need for the CEO to maintain a low profile, to spend time training other people as well as to have the broad experience[2] that gives him a system perspective, suggests a rather mature person who has distinguished himself and who gains satisfaction less from public accolade than from personal achievement. Yet, the job is a particularly stressful one, particularly during the early formative stages, and it is one where the chances of unpopularity are far greater than of popularity.

• While some management methods more appropriate to a system than to an autonomous institution can be taught, others are intuitive and difficult to teach. The findings imply quite strongly that managing a system is complex and requires a broad range of skills.[3] Administrators have traditionally been encouraged to develop a parochial interest in their own organization, but effective system administration requires both broad skills and a broad perspective. In a similar vein, the development of systems also changes the role of the trustee. Data suggests that while skills such as negotiation techniques and process observation can be taught, a system perspective is as difficult to teach as it is to define. Yet if the teaching process is systematic and follows a logical pattern that includes exposure to many kinds of issues, then this too may be taught. Malin, for example, has dealt explicitly with this issue by insisting that his managers have experience that includes menial details as well as the overall capital structure. There certainly is precedence to believe that one can learn to lead; Argyris argues that it can be done by changing one's approach to problem conceptualization and problem resolution. Other people have argued that the way to effectively teach leaders is to pair a learner with an experienced doer and to reward the doer for developing the younger person. Certain companies, among them Jewel and Phillips, have traditionally done this. Of course, the use of mentors is widespread even if it is not necessarily institutionalized. The data suggest that present system leaders have not used this pattern to any significant degree. Perhaps they have felt a need to withhold information until the time for disclosure was appropriate; and, of course, the number of managers in the health sector has been limited. Consequently, the person most likely to be a protégé has traditionally had enough to do in a line or staff position without the added stress of spending non-task-oriented time periods with "the boss." In addition, in order for the mentor-protégé relationship to be successful, the protégé usually needs gradually increased visibility. But the necessary low profile that many system managers choose to keep, at least locally, often excludes such visibility. One answer is to develop someone within the corporate staff who is not viewed as partisan, but this approach implies that the corporate staff is large enough to lose a member. It does little good to "pull" someone out of a job that is viewed as critical for the development of the system, but it could be equally harmful for outsiders to feel that the corporate staff is overstaffed and unnecessarily expensive.

MHSs can be considered to be rapid growth companies (ones that grow at an average rate greater than 20 percent per year). These systems appear to demand an innovative kind of management that uses existing tools but is also willing to discover new ones that are appropriate to the peculiarities of the health system. The CEO needs to make decisions quickly that may have significant consequences, but how will he obtain the necessary data? An application of a "business-oriented" management information system is likely to flood him with data, much of which is not usable. A continuation of the traditional hospital management information system is likely to give him insufficient data. The need for information and the need to diffuse decisions imply significant integration among units; hospitals, even groups of hospitals, have paid little attention to this problem of interrelationships. The need for boundary scanning implies a flexible organizational structure that can obtain and process information. The traditional hospital structure has relied on the CEO to play the major information retrieval and processor role. The system must institutionalize this role. To further complicate the issue, MHSs are so different from autonomous institutions that professional similarities are minimal; the fiscal officer at SSHS has a significantly different job from his counterpart at SJHHS. Consequently, there has been little career advancement among systems.

The particular needs of MHSs imply that the key managers must adapt their attitudes as well as what they actually do to the changing needs of the system. This is not easy to do. A CEO who trained in a hospital may find it difficult to bring young people on board with salaries that seem totally unrealistic and with attitudes that appear to be even less like his own. He may find it difficult to take a broad, analytical perspective and spend time diagnosing where the system is and what it needs to accomplish, and to use other people for jobs that he has traditionally done himself. In fact, the MHS provides a stimulating and challenging environment, one that calls for an innovative and resourceful leader who can use tools that have been developed in private industry and adapt them, as well as his own style, to the changing needs of the developing system.

• The administrator must view his job somewhat differently as a result of system overlap as well as system development. An interesting evolution of the multihospital system is that of contiguous or competing overlapping systems. As these systems begin to encroach on one another's territory and as the performance of one system begins to be used as a benchmark for the other, when historically each system has been able to independently set its own performance standards, an increased level of complexity results that demands a sharing of tasks among systems, rather than among units. The CEOs of such systems must be able to think in an added dimension, and to integrate the many units of these systems. To some extent this is already happening in that SJHHS, SSHS and WAHS are all operating in the same area, but data suggest that this will occur throughout the country as systems enlarge.

It would seem that by understanding and using data about:

the demands of the particular environment
the stage of development through which the system is progressing
the tasks that need to be accomplished and the skills that are useful

the new or experienced manager within a health system can become more effective. Perhaps by comparing the needs of their own systems to those of these seven systems these managers can avoid some of the problems experienced by these systems. If, for example, a particular manager finds himself in a geographically close system, the member units may need to be involved in decision making, and integration may be necessary. Another manager might find himself working in a system that has traditionally depended on a single source of financing, and yet is developing comprehensive programs that suggest long lead times. Based on the data gathered for this book, it would be useful for this system to seek other sources of financing early in the process of program development.

IMPLICATIONS FOR RESEARCHERS

Organizational research has given significant attention to the management of complex systems that operate in conditions of uncertainty, yet little systematic work has been done in the health field. These findings concerning the development of multihospital systems imply that:

• In a health organization, as in other complex structures, an organization's design should fit the environment in which it operates and the goals it wishes to achieve. It would seem that a multihospital system epitomizes a complex system. From an early emphasis on the organization and on methods of scientifically managing people, the field of organizational behavior now emphasizes the people within the organization, particularly ways of enriching the jobs of those people so that their personal satisfaction would lead to overall organizational growth. Now the emphasis within organizational behavior has been on reaching an equilibrium among a number of variables, particularly the environment, the task, and the person.

Researchers and theorists have developed various principles concerning methods of organizing. (These principles are addressed in Chapter 4.) Briefly, they include the contingent use of mechanistic and organic patterns of organizing,[4] the importance of accommodating units to their subenvironments,[5] and the need to buffer uncertainty.[6] While data suggest that there is an important relationship between the level of uncertainty in the environment and the design of the organization, little research has been done on this relationship in the health area. It is in fact surprising how little is known about the environment in which hospitals and other health facilities operate. For this reason, I have found it useful to think of the environment as an "ecological niche," for this term better characterizes the delicate relationship among the various environmental factors and between these factors and the complex system in question. We may now suggest that an awareness of the five environmental variables can expand the literature to be more useful to the specific characteristics of the health sector.

• The role of "leader" in a multihospital system can be divided into a number of necessary tasks that must be performed at different times. Although significant research has been done on the leadership of complex organizations, little work has been done in the health field. While some of the research is of course transferrable, a good deal of it is not because of the peculiar nature of the organizational hierarchy within the hospital. If one were to apply the literature, would one use it to describe the behavior of the CEO, or of the chief medical officer? Both are leaders and in many situations their spheres of control and influence have been unclear.

This book expands on the literature by attempting to fragment the role of the leader into the various visible tasks that he chooses to move the system forward. It also attempts to understand how MHSs develop within environments that are often highly uncertain. The management of such systems appears to be contingent on a number of variables: where the system is in its development determines the tasks that need to be addressed, and the tasks are in turn determined by external demands as well as by internal pressures. It is up to the CEO to diagnose the changing demands of the environment and of the units within the system. It is also up to him to decide which tasks can reasonably be accomplished and which should wait.

IMPLICATIONS FOR THE HEALTH SYSTEM

The proliferation of hospital and multifacility systems has already had a significant impact on the health field, and current as well as forthcoming legislation suggests that this will continue to be true.

• The multihospital systems studied have acquired considerable power by virtue of their ability to purchase staff, technology, and facilities, and consequently to affect the quality of and the accessibility to medical care in a given area, and of national health policy. There is little doubt that health policy has attempted to legislate accessible and appropriate care while at the same time stressing cost containment. But the better the access to care and the broader the range of available services, the higher the cost. For this, as well as for a number of other reasons, planning at the federal level has generally been unsuccessful.

Rather than attempting to legislate changes, the development of systems suggests that the member units can more effectively decide what services should be shared, what services should be unified under one roof and in general, how best to address the needs of a given population. MHSs are well equipped to perform such a planning function; they have the volume, they have the political constituencies, and they often have the managerial and fiscal capability to exert a real impact on the care of a given region. This is not to say that MHSs are the one answer that will rationalize the inequitable and expensive provision of services, but systems do represent one important way of allowing groups of institutions to actively plan rather than reactively adjust to federal legislation.

In terms of the economy of care, the development of systems allows the member institutions access to management capabilities that are likely to be far superior to those they could obtain alone. While small, rural hospitals could hardly be expected to perform complex financial analyses, the rural institutions that make up SJHHS can in fact do so. In addition, a system is able to scan boundaries and forecast the probable effect of changes in the environment far more effectively than the individual hospital, where management tends to be preoccupied with daily crises.

While data concerning cost savings are outside the scope of this book, research does suggest[7] that cost savings can gradually be achieved by developing an effective resource allocation model whereby improved utilization of beds and laboratory facilities are achieved, although such savings remain difficult to measure. This kind of resource allocation model, which takes into account the needs of the patient population, the availability of physicians, and the kind and strength of services, is likely to provide higher quality care at lower prices than the individual institutions could render.

The issue of quality of care is also outside the scope of this book, but it seems logical to assume that by reducing duplication of services, systems are more likely to have better utilized and consequently higher quality facilities.[8] In terms of accessibility of care, it would seem that a system has the luxury of retaining a financially unsound facility because of an overall regional strategy. The ability of a system to secure capital makes this kind of strategy possible. This is not to say that is necessarily a good idea to have a number of financially weak units, but that in terms of an overall strategy that has as an objective to deliver care to a given region, a system might want to retain a critical but "losing" unit. In addition, a system is often free to innovate in terms of the kind of care it provides and thereby improve accessibility. For example, it can begin geriatric units or outreach centers, whereas autonomous hospitals might not have the time available to either plan or staff such innovation.

• The findings of this study imply that the pattern of career development within the health sector may change. Rather than advancing within one institution and then moving on to a more senior position in another institution, the growth of systems implies that a manager could spend the major portion of his career within one system, holding both line and staff jobs. As systems become better known, this kind of manager might become far more attractive than the traditional manager who has made lateral moves without, perhaps, the same depth of experience.

NOTES

1. In his article entitled "Power, Success and Organizational Effectiveness" (*Organizational Dynamics,* Winter 1978), John Kotter points out that while the plant manager of a small plant is dependent on his subordinates, suppliers, markets, and his boss, the head of a teaching hospital depends on the City Council, the Mayor's Office, the City Bureaucracy, numerous unions, the Civil Service, local community groups, other hospitals, the federal government, the local press, the medical school, the state government, and various accreditation agencies.
2. An erroneous assumption has been made that business or educational experience can replace experience gained in the health sector. This has generally proven to be false at the CEO level.
3. A rather unusual image comes to mind here—that of the polo player. To be really competent in this sport, the player has to be so comfortable on the horse that the act of riding need not receive attention as he considers his moves. If he has to think about his capability as a rider, rather than his ability as a polo player, then he can no longer play well. The present or potential administrator of a system has to be so comfortable with the problems of managing an institution that he can concentrate on the issues of system development.
4. Tom Burns and G. M. Stalker, *The Management of Innovation* (London: Tavistock Publications and Social Science Paperback, 1961).
5. Paul R. Lawrence and Jay W. Lorsch, *Organization and Environment* (Boston: Harvard Business School, 1967).
6. James D. Thompson, *Organizations in Action* (New York: McGraw-Hill, 1967).
7. AHA study.
8. It is generally accepted that if, for example, a cardiac surgery team does two coronary bypass procedures a week, its rate of morbidity will be higher than a team that does two each day.

Bibliography

BOOKS

Allen, Stephen A. (1968). *Managing Organizational Diversity.* Boston: Harvard Business School, unpublished doctoral dissertation.

American Hospital Association (1976). *Hospital Statistics.* Chicago: American Hospital Association.

Andrews, Kenneth (1971). *The Concept of Corporate Strategy.* Homewood, Ill.: Dow Jones-Irwin.

Anthony, Robert N., and Regina E. Herzlinger (1975). *Management Control in Nonprofit Organizations.* Homewood, Ill.: Richard D. Irwin, Inc.

Argyris, Chris (1977). *Increasing Leadership Effectiveness.* New York: John Wiley & Sons.

Argyris, Chris, and D. Schon (1974). *Theory in Practice: Increasing Professional Effectiveness.* San Francisco: Jossey-Bass.

Ashby, W. Ross (1964). *An Introduction to Cybernetics.* London: Methuen & Co., Ltd.

Ashby, W. Ross (1965). *Design for a Brain.* London: Chapman & Hall, Ltd., and Science Paperbacks.

Aspen Systems Corporation (1976). *Topics in Health Care Financing: Prospective Rate Setting,* Vol. 3, No. 2, Winter.

Barnard, Chester I. (1938). *The Functions of the Executive.* Cambridge, Mass.: Harvard University Press.

Blake, R. R. (1970). *The Grid for Sales Excellence* (with J. S. Mouton). New York: McGraw-Hill.

171

Brown, Lawrence (1978). *The Formulation of Federal Health Care Policy.* Governmental Studies Program, The Brookings Institution, Washington, D.C., Vol. 54, No. 1, January.

Brown, Montague, and H. Lewis (1976). *Hospital Management Systems.* Germantown, Md.: Aspen Systems Corporation.

Burns, Tom, and G. M. Stalker (1966). *The Management of Innovation,* London: Tavistock Publications and Social Science Paperbacks.

Chandler, Alfred D. (1961). *Strategy and Structure.* Cambridge, Mass.: M.I.T. Press.

Cooney, James P., et al (1975). *Multihospital Systems: An Evaluation. Part 2: Organizational Studies.* Health Services Research Center of the Hospital Research and Educational Trust and Northwestern University.

Cyert, Richard, and James March (1963). *A Behavioral Theory of the Firm.* Englewood Cliffs, N.J.: Prentice-Hall.

Federal Trade Commission (1972). *Conglomerate Merger Performance: An Empirical Study of Nine Corporations.* November.

Fiedler, Fred E. (1967). *A Theory of Leadership Effectiveness.* New York: McGraw-Hill.

Forrester, Jay (1971). *World Dynamics.* Cambridge, Mass.: Wright-Allen Press.

Fuchs, V. R. (1974). *Who Shall Live? Health Economics and Social Choice.* New York: Basic Books.

Galbraith, Jay (1973). *Designing Complex Organizations.* Reading, Mass.: Addison-Wesley.

Georgopoulos, Basil (1975). *Hospital Organization Research: Review and Source.* Philadelphia: Saunders Series in Health Care Organization and Administration.

Harris, Richard (1966). *A Sacred Trust.* New York: New American Library.

Hart, Leslie A. (1975). *How the Brain Works.* New York: Basic Books.

Health Services Research Center of the Hospital Research and Educational Trust and Northwestern University (1975). *Multihospital Systems: An Evaluation.*

Hodgson, R. C., D. J. Levinson, and A. Zaleznick (1965). *The Executive Role Constellation.* Boston: Division of Research, Harvard Business School.

Homans, George (1950). *The Human Group.* New York: Harcourt Brace and Co.

Illich, Ivan (1976). *Medical Nemesis.* New York: Pantheon.

Katz, Daniel, and R. L. Kahn (1966). *The Social Psychology of Organization.* New York: John Wiley & Sons.

Lawrence, Paul R., and Jay W. Lorsch (1967). *Organization and Environment.* Boston: Division of Research, Harvard Business School.

Lawrence, Paul R., and Jay W. Lorsch (1970). *Studies in Organizational Design.* Homewood, Ill.: Irwin & Dorsey.

Levinson, Harry (1968). *The Exceptional Executive.* New York: New American Library.

Lorsch, Jay W., and S. Allen (1973). *Managing Diversity and Interdependence.* Boston: Division of Research, Harvard Business School.

Lynch, Harry H. (1971). *Financial Performance of Conglomerates.* Boston: Division of Research, Harvard Business School.

Mace, Myles, and George Montgomery (1962). *Management Problems of Corporate Acquisitions.* Boston: Division of Research, Harvard Business School.

McGregor, D. (1960). *The Human Side of Enterprise.* New York: McGraw-Hill.

March, James, and Herbert Simon (1958). *Organizations.* New York: John Wiley & Sons.

Mintzberg, Henry (1973). *The Nature of Managerial Work.* New York: Harper & Row.

Moore, Harry (1927). *American Medicine and the People's Health.* New York: D. Appleton.

Mouzelis, Nicos P. (1968). *Organization and Bureaucracy: An Analysis of Modern Theories.* Chicago: Aldine Publishing Co.

National Forum in Hospital and Health Affairs (1975). *A Decade of Implementation: The Multiple Hospital Management Concept Revisited* (report). Duke University.

Newhouse, Joseph P., and Jan Acton (1974). In Clark C. Havighurst, ed., *Regulating Health Facilities Construction.* Washington, D C.: American Enterprise.

Perrow, Charles (1970). *Organizational Analysis: A Sociological View.* London: Tavistock Publications.

Rutstein, David D. (1967). *The Coming Revolution in Medicine.* Cambridge, Mass.: M.I.T. Press.

Schein, Edger H. (1970). *Organizational Psychology.* Englewood Cliffs, N.J.: Prentice-Hall.

Selznick, Philip (1957). *Leadership in Administration.* New York: Harper & Row.

Somers, Anne (1971). *Health Care in Transition: Directions for the Future,* Chicago: Hospital Research and Educational Trust.

Steiner, Peter O. (1975). *Mergers.* Ann Arbor: University of Michigan Press.

Thompson, James D. (1967). *Organizations in Action.* New York: McGraw-Hill.

Touche, Ross (1976). *Health Care Horizons 1976.* Forty-fourth Annual Review of Hospital Operations.

Touche, Ross (1977). *Health Care Horizons 1977.* Forty-fifth Annual Review of Hospital Operations.

Ward, Richard A. (1975). *The Economics of Health Resources.* Reading, Mass.: Addison-Wesley.

Weber, Max (1947). *The Theory of Social and Economic Organization.* New York: The Free Press,

Wilson, Florence, and Duncan Neuhauser (1974). *Health Services in the United States.* Cambridge, Mass.: Ballinger.

Woodward, Joan (1965). *Industrial Organization: Theory and Practice.* London: Oxford University Press.

ARTICLES, MONOGRAPHS, CASES

Argyris, Chris (1973). "The CEO's Behavior: Key to Organizational Development," *Harvard Business Review* 51, March–April.
Bales, R. (1954). "In Conference." *Harvard Business Review*, March–April.
Berry, Ralph (1974). "Perspectives on Rate Regulation" (monograph), in *Controls on Health Care, Institute of Medicine.* Washington, D.C.: National Academy of Sciences.
Boston Medical and Surgical Journal 1, no. 399 (1968). "Duties of Hospital Physicians and Surgeons."
Brown, Jonothan, and Marc Roberts (1977). "Health Care Expenditures Since 1950" (monograph). Boston: Harvard School of Public Health.
Brown, Montague (1978). "Changing Role of the Administrator in Multiple Hospital Systems," *Hospital and Health Services Administration*, Fall.
Brown, Montague, and William H. Money (1975). "The Promise of Multihospital Management," *Hospital Progress*, August–September.
Brown, Montague, and William H. Money (1976). "Contract Management: Is It for Your Hospital?" *Trustee* 29, February.
Business Week (1974). "Why the Nation's Hospitals May Well Go Broke," October 26.
Business Week (1975). "Performing Major Surgery on Hospital Costs," May 19.
Christenson, Charles (1973). "The 'Contingency Theory' of Organizations: A Methodological Analysis." Boston: Harvard Business School, Working Paper #73–36.
Curran, William J., J. Steel, and E. W. Ober (1975). "Government Intervention on the Increase," *Hospitals* 49:10, May 16.
Curran, William J. (1970). "Health Planning Agencies: A Legal Crisis?" *American Journal of Public Health* 60:2, February.
Curran, William J. (1976). "Present at the Creation: Health Planning and the Inevitable Reorganization," *Health Care Management Review*, Winter.
Daedalus (1977). "Journal of the Academy of Arts and Sciences: Doing Better and Feeling Worse" (monograph), Winter.
Densen, Paul, and Katharine Bauer (1973). *Some Issues in the Incentive Reimbursement Approach to Cost Containment: An Overview.* Boston: Harvard Center for Community Health and Medical Care, May.
DeVries, Robert A. (1978). "Health Care Delivery: Strength in Numbers," *Hospitals* 52, March 16.
Doody, Michael F. (1974). "Status on Multihospital Systems," *Hospitals* 48, June 1.
Duncan, Robert B. (1972). "Characteristics of Organizational Environments and Perceived Environmental Uncertainty," *Administrative Science Quarterly* 17.
Elling, R. H., and S. Halebsky (1961). "Organizational Differentiation and Support," *Administrative Science Quarterly* 6:2.
Ehrbar, A. F. (1977). "A Radical Prescription for Medical Care," *Fortune*, February.

Enthoven, A., and R. Noll, "Regulatory and Non-Regulatory Strategies for Controlling Health Care Costs" (monograph). Stanford University, Research Paper #402, September.

Fein, Rashi (1975). "Some Health Policy Issues: One Economist's View," *Public Health Reports* 90:5, September–October.

Feldstein, M., and A. Taylor (1977). "The Rapid Rise of Hospital Costs." Council on Wage and Price Stability, Executive Office of the President, January.

Fiedler, Fred E., Victor H. Vroom, and Chris Argyris (1977). *Organizational Dynamics: Leadership Symposium*. American Management Association.

Fortune (1977). "A Radical Perspective," February.

Friedson, Elliot (ed.) (1963). "Goals and Power Structures," in *The Hospital in Modern Society*. New York: The Free Press.

Hallen, Philip B. (1963). "Hospitals Branch-Out: A Study of Multiple Unit Operations," *Hospitals* 37, August 1, Part I.

Harvey, N. A. (1965). "Cybernetic Applications in Medicine I. Medical Model Making," *New York Journal of Medicine,* March 15.

Heller, Karen S. (1976). "Approaches to Health Planning and Regulation in the United States: A Review." Boston: Harvard School of Public Health.

Kennedy, Senator E. (1971), in U.S. Congress. "Health Care Crisis in America, Part I." Hearings before the Subcommittee on Health, 92nd Congress, First Session, February 23.

Klicka, Karl S. (1967). "Managing a Multiple-Unit Hospital System," *Hospitals* 41, October 16.

Krause, Elliot (1973). "Health Planning as a Managerial Ideology," *International Journal of Health Services* 3.

Lawrence, Paul R., and Jay W. Lorsch (1976b). "New Management Job: The Integrator," *Harvard Business Review* 45, November–December.

Malm, H. M. (1974). "Multi-Hospital Management, Analyzing and Example," *Hospital Administration,* Spring.

Mecklin, John M. (1970). "Hospitals Need Management Even More Than Money," *Fortune,* January.

Modern Hospital (1973). "Looking Around: The Multiple Hospital is the Only Way to Go," November.

Osler, William (1908). "Remarks on the Functions of an Outpatient Department," *British Medical Journal,* June 20.

Pave, Irene (1977). "The 9% Flaw in Carter's Hospital Plan," *Business Week,* May 9.

Platou, Carl N., and James A. Rice (1972). "Multihospital Holding Companies," *Harvard Business Review,* May–June.

Posner, Richard A. (1974). "Certificate of Need for Health Care Facilities Construction: A Dissenting View." In *Regulating Health Care Facilities Construction,* edited by C. V. Havighurst. Washington, D.C.: American Enterprise Institute for Public Policy Research.

Rohrer, W. C. (1962). "Demographic and Social Changes Affecting the Community Hospital," *Hospital Administration* 7:3.

Scott, Bruce R. (1972). *Stages of Corporate Development: A Descriptive Model* (monograph). Boston: Harvard Business School, ICCH #13G372.

Sheldon, Alan, and Diana Barrett (1977). "The Janus Principle," *Health Care Management Review,* Spring.

Silver, Arnold P., and Samandar M. Hai (1977). *Report on the Task Force on Measuring and Financing Working Capital Needs for Hospitals: A Summary.* Prepared for Principles and Practices Board, Hospital Financial Management Association, February.

Tannenbaum, R., and W. Schmidt (1973). "How to Choose a Leadership Pattern," *Harvard Business Review,* May–June.

Toomey, R. (1977). "County Facilities Equitably Serve All Residents," *Hospitals* 51, March 1.

Trevelyan, Eoin (1973). *Fairview Community Hospitals* (A) (case), Boston: Harvard Business School, ICCH #9-374-001.

Trevelyan, Eoin (1973). *Fairview Community Hospitals* (B) (case), Boston: Harvard Business School, ICCH #9-374-002.

Trustee (1976). "Multihospital Systems: The Older They Get, the Better They Run," December.

United States Department of Health, Education, and Welfare (1977). *The Priorities of Section 1502.* Papers on the National Guidelines, Public Health Service, Health Resources Administration.

Vroom, Victor H. (1973). "A New Look at Managerial Decision-Making," *Organizational Dynamics,* Spring.

Index

About the Author

Diana Barrett received her M.B.A. and D.B.A. from Harvard Business School. She is on the faculty of the Harvard School of Public Health, where she teaches organizational behavior and strategy implementation. Dr. Barrett has had extensive experience as a consultant in the health field, particularly in the areas of organizational strategy and program development. Her clients have included private and public teaching hospitals as well as smaller community hospitals and other health care providers who find themselves in a rapidly changing environment that makes new demands on them and often leads to collaborative arrangements. Dr. Barrett also lectures extensively on the problems of establishing various kinds of multihospital systems.